The Hospice Companion

The Hospice Companion

Second Edition

Best Practices for Interdisciplinary
Assessment and Care of Common
Problems During the Last Phase of Life

Perry G. Fine, MD

Professor of Anesthesiology
Pain Research Center
School of Medicine
University of Utah
Salt Lake City, Utah

Associate Editor

Matthew Kestenbaum, MD

Chief of the Medical Staff
Capital Caring
Washington, DC

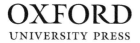

OXFORD
UNIVERSITY PRESS

OXFORD
UNIVERSITY PRESS

Oxford University Press, Inc., publishes works that further
Oxford University's objective of excellence
in research, scholarship, and education.

Oxford New York
Auckland Cape Town Dar es Salaam Hong Kong Karachi
Kuala Lumpur Madrid Melbourne Mexico City Nairobi
New Delhi Shanghai Taipei Toronto

With offices in
Argentina Austria Brazil Chile Czech Republic France Greece
Guatemala Hungary Italy Japan Poland Portugal Singapore
South Korea Switzerland Thailand Turkey Ukraine Vietnam

Published by Oxford University Press, Inc.
198 Madison Avenue, New York, New York 10016
www.oup.com

Oxford is a registered trademark of Oxford University Press

Library of Congress Cataloging-in-Publication Data
The hospice companion : best practices for interdisciplinary assessment and care of
common problems during the last phase of life / [edited by] Perry G. Fine ; associate
editor, Matthew Kestenbaum.—2nd ed.
p. ; cm.
Rev. ed of: The hospice companion / Perry G. Fine. 2008.
Includes bibliographical references and index.
ISBN 978-0-19-984079-3
I. Fine, P. G. (Perry G.) II. Kestenbaum, Matthew. III. Fine, P. G. (Perry G.) Hospice
companion.
[DNLM: 1. Hospice Care—methods—Handbooks. 2. Palliative Care—methods—
Handbooks. 3. Patient Care Team—Handbooks. 4. Terminally Ill—psychology—
Handbooks. WB 39]
LC Classification not assigned
362.17'56—dc23
2011053131

9 8 7 6 5

Printed in the United States of America
on acid-free paper

Acknowledgments

This second edition of *The Hospice Companion* reflects labors of love by the entire staff of Capital Caring, a premier advanced illness coordinated health-care system providing hospice and palliative care services throughout the metropolitan Washington DC area. Their work is possible only due to the visionary and courageous leadership of this organization's Chief Executive Officer, Malene Davis: visionary, because of her foresight to see the necessity of high-quality comprehensive services that extend far beyond the last days of life for people living with chronic progressive illnesses; courageous, because of her willingness to go at risk, break away from conventional and limited models of care, insist on measuring what matters most, *never* deny needed care to *anyone* for *any* reason, support education for the next generation of hospice and palliative medicine specialists, partner with traditional health-care systems in novel and innovative ways, develop a research enterprise to advance the field, and prove that this can and must be done within a sustainable economic model. And last, but far from least, we are immeasurably grateful for the trust of the many families who open their doors to us each and every day, and allow us the privilege of being of service, which propels us ever forward in our individual and collective evolution as a civil society—where each of us is stronger for the dignity we help each other achieve throughout the entirety of our lives.

Foreword

Medical anthropologists of the future may look back at the start of the American hospice benefit with both amazement at its prescience and bemusement at the problems that its structure was predestined to pose. When first established, it was an extraordinary innovation, a leap of faith that a model of home-based palliative care could be created and sustained in a complex and fragmented health-care system focused relentlessly on the curing of disease. The outcome of this leap has been clear for many years: Hospice has been a roaring success during the more than quarter-century since it began. Looking to the future, it is both this success and acknowledgement of its problems that can help chart the path forward into an era of health-care reform in the United States.

Advocates, policymakers, and clinicians, working from knowledge of a novel care model in the United Kingdom but with no blueprint for the larger U.S. health system, proposed a new government entitlement that was ultimately codified in the Tax Equity and Fiscal Responsibility Act of 1982. It offered a program that potentially would be available to millions, and through conditions of participation for certified agencies, effectively operationalized a system for palliative care at the end of life. This accomplishment is truly stunning when the context of the time is appreciated: It was developed without a uniformly accepted definition of palliative care, without knowledge of the elements of specialist care that would evolve in the decades thereafter, and without a historical precedent for a payment model that could sustain coordinated interdisciplinary care and associated services. It used the compelling desire to improve the U.S. system's ability to provide for a "good death" at home to fashion a system that, perhaps unintentionally, promoted an emerging vision of a broader model of palliative care. Through a new regulatory framework, it required providers to focus on patients with advanced illnesses and their families, and develop an integrated system of meetings and reports capable of coordinating interventions that reduce suffering and illness burden, and support the values and preferences of the patient and family.

The hospice benefit was created in a fee-for-service environment to support comprehensive care, much of which was non-reimbursable. It did this by becoming the country's first managed-care plan, predicated on per diem reimbursement for an agency's full-risk assumption of expense related to the terminal illness. Remarkably, this approach foreshadowed the key principle of risk sharing that has been incorporated into many of the health-care reform strategies looming in the United States.

Hospice has evolved into one of the best benefits in health care, and it is no surprise that the program has grown dramatically since it began. Eligible patients and families obtain professional services, volunteer services, access to inpatient care, drugs, supplies, equipment, bereavement services, and other interventions related to the terminal illness, and do so without co-pay, without deductible, and without the need for co-insurance. Hospice services generate the highest satisfaction ratings among families exposed to different systems of care.

Hospice now serves more than 1 million Medicare patients annually—more than 40% of Medicare beneficiaries who die each year—and the annual cost to the government of this care is now more than $12 billion. With strong evidence that the overall costs for patients receiving the hospice benefit are far less than comparable patients receiving routine care, this expenditure is, on balance, as good for the system as it is for the patients and families it affects. Even as the government takes action to address the economic disparities in the industry and the possibility that excessive opportunities for profit may exist in some areas, the overall conclusion remains unchanged: Hospice reduces the high cost inherent in the care of patients with progressive incurable illness nearing the end of life, and this, as much as the quality of care, should be a key driver for broader adoption.

The problems and concerns about hospice, many of which were prefigured by decisions made at the time that the benefit was created, do not negate these positives, but do present opportunities for improvement. Regrettably, hospice was built as a separate health system outside of mainstream medicine. It was linked inextricably to death and dying through eligibility that required prognostication of life expectancy. It fixed payments at per diem rates irrespective of treatments that may still be appropriate for the disease. It did not require hospice-employed physicians to see patients, and although it regulated the elements of care, it did not build in the requirement to evaluate quality of care delivery.

Each of these aspects poses challenges. With a system constructed outside of mainstream medicine, and with limited involvement of physicians, it is understandable that physicians generally, and other health professionals as well, have an unacceptable knowledge gap about eligibility for the benefit or the services it offers. With eligibility tied to dying, rather than the need for care, and requiring a degree of future prognostication that is clearly beyond medical capability, it is not surprising that late referrals are the rule and that physicians and others often communicate inaccurately about the benefit. Professionals, patients and families, and the lay public all appear to view this program as a system to assist the actively dying, rather than as a comprehensive set of home-based services that can reduce the burden of illness for both patients and families when illness is advanced. With the reluctance of Americans—including patients and professionals—to discuss dying, even the mention of hospice may be reserved to a point very late on the trajectory of disease. Delay in referral also may be determined by the payment model, which provides for no additional revenues when patients are still appropriately receiving expensive disease-modifying therapies. The inability to assume these costs leads to the conclusion that "aggressive" treatments are outside of the hospice's scope of practice, and communication about these limitations back to the referring community helps solidify the perspective that referral to hospice is appropriate only when disease-modifying treatments have ended and death is anticipated very soon.

With the remarkable and positive changes that have occurred in the hospice industry during decades of growth, with the emergence of palliative care specialists in many disciplines and palliative care consultation programs in most hospitals, and with the anticipation of enormous change coming in the healthcare system, hospice is poised to expand its influence and contributions to American health care. To do so, hospice agencies must understand that they represent the United States' key resource for the provision of specialist-level home-based palliative care for patients with advanced illness. They will need to support the training and professionalism of staff; develop closer alignment with physicians, hospitals, nursing homes, and home care agencies; and drive the focus on quality.

The training of staff is essential, and from this perspective, accolades are due the work of Fine and Kestenbaum in *The Hospice Companion*. Accessible, state-of-the-art materials for education and training of hospice professionals like this one must be disseminated and used to support performance improvement.

Hospice has been an extraordinarily successful model that has positively influenced the palliative care movement in the United States, the effort to bring comprehensive patient-centered care to the broader management of the chronically ill, and the use of shared risk assumption as a means to provide cost-effective care. It promises to continue this influence in the emerging era of health reform.

Russell Portenoy, MD
Chairman and Gerald J. Friedman Chair
in Pain Medicine and Palliative Care
Department of Pain Medicine and Palliative Care
Beth Israel Medical Center
and
Chief Medical Officer
MJHS Hospice and Palliative Care
and
Professor of Neurology and Anesthesiology
Albert Einstein College of Medicine

Preface

Almost 30 years ago, with the stroke of a pen, one of the most remarkable developments in modern health care occurred: the enactment of the Medicare Hospice Benefit. This public policy development was an acknowledgment that hospital-based care for the dying was discordant with essential human needs at this unique time in the life cycle and that there was a reasonable economic alternative. But for just as long, I have called this "the best-kept secret in American health care" because still, after three decades, far too few people—including doctors as well as patients and their loved ones—understand the extraordinary value of this all-inclusive service: value that can be measured both in terms of well-defined and highly desirable clinical outcomes and dollars. After the fact, those who do obtain hospice care often ask, "Why didn't we learn about this earlier?" It's a good question, and one whose answer lies in cultural change. Even though more and more people with life-limiting diseases are connecting with hospice care, there remain hundreds of thousands who die in the United States without the benefit of hospice's focus on comfort, family support, and dignity. The initial conception of *The Hospice Companion* was spurred by comparing the scientific and structured approach that is the hallmark of modern medicine and the heartfelt and often spiritually driven paradigm of hospice care. In my observations of how dying patients were treated in hospital settings, the former seemed to lack "heart," but conversely community-based hospice care seemed to lack the rigor of measured self-inspection. Both are necessary; neither is sufficient to attend to the toll that advanced illness takes on the body, mind, and spirit. Both are needed, and since most of us want to complete our lives in familiar surroundings (wherever we call "home"), and because the acute care model of the contemporary hospital is both anathema to the optimal end-of-life experience as well as inordinately expensive, I submit that there is no reason why "hospice heart" and "hospice mind" cannot be fostered and intertwined. Yet empirically based scientific advancements and salutary minimization of unwarranted variability in clinical care delivery—especially around pain and symptom management—has been slow to develop within hospice. Bridging this divide was the motivation for publishing the first edition of *The Hospice Companion*.

It was therefore heartening that Oxford University Press reported the need for a reprinting of the book. But as gratifying as it was to hear that the manual was being used, it unleashed in me a potent storm of multiple and seemingly paradoxical neurotransmitter releases because of the publisher's concomitant request for a second edition—and soon! (I hope that you appreciate my attempt at humor here, realizing it is a rarity when one can use such a phrase—"multiple and seemingly paradoxical neurotransmitter releases"—with a straight face, and that humor is what fortifies us in the often harrowing circumstances we face in our work). By use of this pharmacologic allusion,

I mean that dopaminergic (euphoria!), sympathetic (excitement!), and cholinergic (run for the restroom!) pathways were simultaneously activated. Those sparking receptors corresponded to my enthusiastic reaction at the culmination of my aspiration to see hospice move toward a more disciplined and structured approach without losing its "soul." If hospice practitioners saw worth in *The Hospice Companion*, it said to me that they saw worth in the approach it promulgated and taught, in order to more effectively meet the needs of people facing the burdens of severe illness and death—and to be able to prove it to a skeptical world with something more substantial than anecdote. This, other than purely financial drivers (which can work for or against rational change), is a powerful impetus for the cultural shift we need. However, that concomitant dysphoric queasiness could only signal the uncontrollable reaction that comes with the demands of a major rewrite in a narrow timeframe!

Speaking of humor, a fellowship-trained, board-certified hospice physician walks into a bar with a gorgeous parrot on her shoulder. The bartender exclaims, "Wow! That certainly is a rare bird?!" To which the parrot responds, "You can say that again!" And so it came to me; hospice is most certainly a "team sport." And I had an extraordinary team in my midst: the medical staff of Capital Caring. This is the largest "flock of rare birds" working together as an organized group of specialists in advanced illness coordinated care that I know of. Through their collective efforts, under the apt and shepherding eye of chief of staff Dr. Matt Kestenbaum, we have been able to research, update, and improve this edition in record time—while salving my autonomic nervous system! In this edition, we have updated the largest section of the manual, pertaining to clinical processes and symptom management. This is where most changes influencing clinical practice have occurred over the past several years, and it is our intent to ensure that hospice professionals stay abreast of advances in the field. As such, each chapter now concludes with a list of recommended readings, culled from the complete literature searches that were done for each symptom complex.

We trust that you will find credibility and authority in the recommendations put forth in this manual, and that it serves you well in your professional role, enhancing your knowledge, skills, and confidence. But in the end, it is our deep and abiding hope that reference to the 2nd edition of *The Hospice Companion* will markedly and measurably improve the lives of those who entrust their care to you. The ironic truism enumerated in the Foreword to the first edition bears repetition: "It will be through disciplined clinical conformity and uniformity of practice that individual epiphany may have the chance to be realized as we meet our earthly ends."

Thank you for your service, your commitment, your fealty—to your profession and to your fellow man.

Perry G. Fine, MD

362.1756
F4938h

Contents

4. Appendices

Contributors

Farrah Daly, MD
Hospice Medical Director
Capital Caring
Leesburg, VA
Chapter: Seizures

Amit Desai, DO
Hospice Medical Director
Capital Caring
Washington, DC
Chapter: Constipation

Ray Jay Garcia, MD
Hospice Medical Director
Capital Caring
Arlington, VA
Chapter: Skin Breakdown: Prevention and Treatment

Jennie GilBhrighde, MD
Physician Fellow
National Institutes of Health/
Capital Caring
Bethesda, MD/Falls
Church, VA
Chapter: Bleeding, Oozing, and Malodorous Lesions

Hunter Groninger, MD
Staff Clinician, Pain and Palliative Care Clinical Center
National Institutes of Health
Bethesda, MD
Chapter: Urinary Problems

Matthew Irwin, MD, MSW
Hospice Medical Director
Capital Caring
Alexandria, VA
Chapter: Air Hunger (Dyspnea)

Natalie Kontakos, MD
Hospice Medical Director
Capital Caring
Alexandria, VA
Chapter: Agitation and Anxiety

Matthew Kestenbaum, MD
Chief, Medical Staff
Capital Caring
Falls Church, VA
Chapter: Anorexia and Cachexia

Dona Leskuski, DO
Hospice Medical Director
Capital Caring
Washington, DC
Chapter: Dysphagia and Oropharyngeal Problems

Jay Lippman, MD
Hospice Medical Director
Capital Caring
Washington, DC
Chapter: Insomnia and Nocturnal Restlessness

Cameron Muir, MD
Executive Vice President
of Quality
and Access
Capital Caring
Falls Church, VA
Chapter: Imminent Death

Alvin Reaves, MD
Physician Fellow
National Institutes of Health/
Capital Caring
Bethesda, MD/Falls Church, VA
Chapter: Fever and Diaphoresis

Marilyn Lewis Renfield, MD

Clinical Assistant Professor of
Psychiatry and Child Development
George Washington University
School of Medicine
Washington, DC
and
Consultant Physician
Capital Caring
Falls Church, VA
Chapter: Depression

Amjad Riar, MD

Hospice Medical Director
Capital Caring
Leesburg, VA
*Chapters: Hiccups; Pain; Skeletal
Muscle and Bladder Spasms*

Randy Schisler, MD

Physician Fellow
National Institutes of Health/
Capital Caring
Bethesda, MD/Falls Church, VA
*Chapters: Belching and Burping
(Eructation); Coughing*

James Shear, MD

Hospice Medical Director
Capital Caring
Alexandria, VA
Chapter: Nausea and Vomiting

Muhammad Siddiqui, MD

Hospice Medical Director
Capital Caring
Falls Church, VA
Chapter: Pruritus

Anne Silao-Solomon, MD

Hospice Medical Director
Capital Caring
Leesburg, VA
Chapter: Confusion/Delirium

Malgorzata Sullivan, MD

Hospice Medical Director
Capital Caring
Washington, DC
Chapter: Xerostomia

Richard Travers, MD

Hospice Physician
Capital Caring
Manassas, VA
*Chapter: Diarrhea and Anorectal
Problems*

Richard Weinberg, MD

Hospice Medical Director
Capital Caring
Falls Church, VA
*Chapter: Fatigue, Weakness
(Aesthenia), and Excessive
Sedation*

Ivan Zama, MD

Hospice Medical Director
Capital Caring
Largo, MD
*Chapter: Edema: Peripheral Edema,
Ascites, and Lymphedema*

Section 1

General Processes

Palliative Care at the End of Life: Blending Structure and Function

From Information to Care

The overarching purpose of this manual, reflecting the essential goals of hospice, is to help maximize the quality of living and dying of patients during the last phase of life. With due regard for the complexities of peoples' lives, especially during severe illness, it is premised that identification and understanding of discrete situations (intertwined and enmeshed as they may be) will promote the elaboration of a care plan that will have the greatest likelihood of meeting these worthy ends.

A sequential system of reasoning and problem-solving is required, and this has been devised using a standardized format throughout each subsection related to symptom management (Section Three). To accommodate the interdisciplinary nature of hospice care and promote use of this manual by all members of the interdisciplinary team (IDT), headings have purposefully been chosen that reflect a common language for all disciplines. In full appreciation of the complex and irreducible nature of human dying, an organized structure is nonetheless useful to define the mechanics and fundamentals of hospice care and the overall goal of making high-quality interdisciplinary care during the last phase of life the rule, rather than the exception.

The overall schema is summarized below. This is followed by an elaboration of terms and concepts used throughout *The Hospice Companion*.

It is recognized that variables such as advanced stage of disease at the time of hospice admission, often with very short survival times, may severely curtail the range of services that might otherwise be useful to patients and families if they had the benefit of an earlier referral with a resultant longer length of stay. In many cases, the processes of care in this book might appear to be idealized because so many patients are referred to hospice just before they die. Therefore, the full range of evaluation, assessment, and interventions proposed may need to be changed in order to hone in on the highest priorities of the patient and family to meet their most pressing needs before death. At the time of admission, attention to the likely longevity of the patient (i.e., prognosis) needs to be well considered so that the issues and goals elaborated in this guide might be realistically and specifically tailored to the needs and attainable goals of each and every patient.

The flow chart "Basic Steps: Taking Care of People Who Are Dying, and Doing It Well" (Figure 1.1) depicted in this section defines the essential steps

Evaluation/Assessment
- Tools- history (all sources, including past medical records) (80% of overall time/effort)
    - physical exam (15+% of overall time/effort)
    - labs, imaging, other tests (<5% of overall time/effort)

Understanding
- Patient
- Context of Patient and Family
- Family

Articulation and Documentation of Realistic/Attainable Goals Taking into Account Major Stakeholders' Needs, Requirements and Expectations
- Patient
- Family
- System
    - referring physician
    - payer
    - patient's healthcare network or system

Development of Care Plan: First the Patient, Then the Family
- Physical Symptoms
- Practical Needs
- PsychoSocial and Spiritual Needs

Everything We Do is an Intervention (for more detailed information, see Section B. below)

Medical	**Non-Medical**	
- Additional Evaluation	- Practical Care	➡ **Defines Staffing** Requirements
- Diagnosis/Prognosis	- Interdisciplinary Team Care	(i.e., Human Resources, FTEs)
- Procedures/Prescriptions for symptom management		

Thoughtful Consideration of Benefits and Burdens Anticipated and/or Resulting from Our Interventions: Discuss These at the Interdisciplinary Team Meeting

Outcomes
- Measurement and Documentation of Outcomes of Interventions
- Analysis of Results

Refine, Revisit, Reassess, Improve
- Is the plan working? If not, why not? How can this be remedied?

Reiterate the Process, Revising the Plan of Care Around the Goal of Optimizing the Following Quality of Life Domains and End-Outcome Measures

- QOL Domains
    - Physical symptoms and functions
    - Intrapersonal dimensions (eg, mood, sense of hope)
    - Interpersonal status (eg, relationships)
    - Transcendent issues (eg, sence of meaning)
- Outcomes
    - Safe and comfortable dying
    - Self-determined life closure
    - Effective coping with imminent loss/bereavement

Figure 1.1 Basic steps of how to care for people who are dying: A logical progression of hospice case management

that need to be followed, or at least considered, in the process of caring for patients at the end of life. It also serves as a teaching tool and reminder of the fundamental goals of patient-centered care within a larger system of health care. Last, it should help unravel the complex nature of the care system, clearly defining steps along the way that lead to successful patient outcomes and professional gratification.

The role of hospice is to deliver the most effective end-of-life care in the most efficient manner possible to all dying patients.

Principles of Effective Care

- The patient defines what help is needed and wanted. However, counseling about what is possible and realizable is critically important because many patients and families will be unaware of the scope of hospice services.
- As a hospice professional, know what you can contribute to accomplish these goals.
- Know who to call upon when you reach the limits of your capabilities.
- Think and act positively. "Can't" or "Won't" is not helpful.
- Actively listen: this is a powerful tool for understanding others, validating peoples' needs to be understood, and planning and providing care.
- Define *benefits* and *burdens* for each proposed therapeutic intervention (note: advising, counseling, and taking a "watch-and-wait" approach are all forms of an "intervention" and in this vein should be viewed in equal regard as medical treatments), remembering that there are distinct points of view: patient, family, other caregivers, professional staff, and other "stakeholders" (e.g., payers]). Ask and answer: What is each party hoping for? What are the underlying motivations?
- *Benefits* and *burdens* are context-driven, requiring a full understanding of each patient's clinical and social circumstances. Determine in advance how benefits and burdens will be assessed, how often, and by whom. If *burdens* can be anticipated (e.g., constipation from an opioid analgesic), how can they be minimized in order to amplify benefits?
- Set priorities by determining which issues are most pressing.

Principles of Efficient Care

- Time is the most precious commodity we have. It must be allocated wisely and well.
- More goods (durable medical equipment, supplies, drugs), in and of themselves, do not equal better service or care. Determine what and how much of these items are necessary to accomplish the patient's goals, and continually reevaluate if they are doing what is intended.
- Clinical managers/leaders should cross-train and schedule human resources wisely. Determine how members of the IDT can meet patient/family goals, both to utilize their unique skills and to distribute work in an equitable and optimal fashion.

Terminology and Organizational Elements Used in Sections 2 and 3 of This Manual

Sections 2 and 3 of this manual will be structured in a similar manner as a means of reinforcing interdisciplinary, comprehensive care. Depending upon relevance, most, but not all, sections will include every dimension of assessment and process of care.

Situation

Every patient/family comes to hospice with unique attributes, clinical circumstances, and social contexts. The process of elucidating those situations that affect the well-being of each patient/family is critical to the provision of good care.

Causes

Most troublesome situations encountered by hospice patients/families can be traced to a single dominant cause or multiple contributory causes. These causes usually stem from one or more of the following domains:

- Practical (i.e., environmental, financial)
- Biomedical (i.e., disease-induced or treatment-related etiology)
- Psychosocial (i.e., related to interpersonal or intrapersonal issues)
- Spiritual (although not always easily defined in words, spiritual concerns often revolve around issues of one's sense of purpose, existence, or meaningfulness, in life and after death)

For the purposes of this guide, causes will be identified for those medically induced symptoms for which a differential diagnosis is important in the consideration of medically specific treatments.

These listings of causes are not meant to be all-inclusive but rather to provide the leading or first-line and secondary causes for most symptoms.

Findings

Findings are those elements (usually *symptoms* [patient report] and *signs* [information obtained by observation or examination]) that define or accompany any given situation and may help to identify the cause(s) of that situation. Findings are also categorized as Practical, Biomedical/Physical, Psychosocial, or Spiritual. These findings serve to identify, direct, and focus processes of care.

Assessment

The initial and ongoing determinations of Psychosocial, Biomedical/Physical, and Spiritual findings involve information-gathering from one or more of the following three basic domains:

- History

Information obtainable from all sources (medical records, interviews with patient, family members, other caregivers) is far and away the most time-consuming and important part of evaluation.

- Physical Examination

This component of assessment involves observation of patient, family and environment, and hands-on examination of the patient. Albeit essential for accurate diagnosis, physical examination also links the patient and caregiver through human touch, which has therapeutic value in and of itself. Needless to say, only skilled and appropriately licensed clinicians should be involved in physical examination of the patient.

- Diagnostic Studies (blood work, imaging, other)

These types of corroborative studies are often unnecessary in order to provide high-quality palliative care at the end of life; however, there are circumstances where clinical impressions derived from history and physical examination are insufficient to formulate a well-conceived care plan. Under these circumstances, the potential benefits need to be weighed against the actual or likely burdens.

Processes of Care
The interventions listed within this section define those actions that might be taken by the IDT in order to meet patient/family needs and goals, identified through sufficient assessment.

Goals and Outcomes
Establishing goals at the outset aligns the patient/family/hospice team and promotes the monitoring of the most relevant outcomes. By explicitly stating goals, the IDT can continually assess the value of the work being done, and determine if the Plan of Care is appropriate. Anticipation of eventualities and putting contingency plans into place are critically important to delivering high-quality end-of-life care. Ideally, outcomes will match the goals that are identified. In other words, the closer outcomes are to goals, the more successful hospice care has been.

Documentation and Medical Record
Guidance is provided in the crucial areas of Initial Assessment, Interdisciplinary Team Notes, and IDT Care Plan in order to promote concise and pertinent record keeping. Thoughtful consideration of what needs to be documented serves the dual purposes of meeting regulatory compliance standards and helping the IDT to continually rethink and revisit issues that arise or are likely to arise in the context of any given patient/family system.

The Practical, Biomedical, Psychological, and Spiritual Dimensions of the Human Experience
The many inseparable dimensions of the human experience cannot be so readily categorized or unintegrated, especially under the circumstances of facing the end of one's life. As important as it may be to acknowledge this, it is equally important to identify and meet the various needs and attainable goals of dying patients and their families, with the hope that each individual can find meaning and value in his or her life as that life comes to a close. From this pragmatic starting point, four axes, or dimensions, have been used in *The Hospice Companion* to sort out and understand the nature of FINDINGS, ASSESSMENT, and PROCESSES OF CARE. **It is critically important for the IDT to understand that these dimensions do not delineate lines of inquiry or intervention by specific disciplines but rather those facets of the patient's or family's experience for which discrete aspects of the Care Plan can be formulated and carried out and outcomes can be measured.**

Practical

These are the everyday, fundamentally important things that surround our lives, most of which we take for granted while we are healthy and able to care for ourselves.

Biomedical

This aspect of end-of-life care addresses the impact of disease on the human body and those tools that modify, reverse, slow, or palliate the progression/consequences of these inevitable biological processes. A depth of clinical knowledge, judgment, and experience is needed to understand and appropriately apply modern medical interventions in ways that will best serve the various needs and goals of patients at this stage in their life.

Psychosocial

Psychological, emotional, and social issues constitute the intrapersonal and interpersonal nature of human existence. These issues are highly complex even under the least stressful circumstances and become the focus of most need once basic physical symptoms are brought under control. Attention to these issues in ways that speak to the needs of dying patients and their families is implicit to quality hospice care.

Spiritual

Ultimately, one's sense of connection, meaning, purpose, or value within the greater scheme of things is most likely to rise to the surface when confronting mortality. Attention to this uniquely human concern, at the pace and within the framework of the patient/family ethos, presents a truly marvelous opportunity for everyone involved and distinguishes hospice care from other alternatives within the health-care system.

Balancing Benefits and Burdens of All Interventions

Because assessment and treatment approaches offer a mixture of possible benefits and burdens to the patient, which vary depending upon each patient's circumstances, considerable thought is needed to attend the best means to optimize benefits, while minimizing burdens. The following stepwise outline should facilitate this process (see Figure 1.2).

First

Prior to all medical procedures, all psychosocial or diagnostic tests, prescriptions, and spiritual care interventions:

- Review pathophysiology and prognosis of ongoing disease.
- Review family structure, support, beliefs, culture, and community ties.
- Review options for palliation of symptoms tailored to the medical/social context of the patient.
- Consider comorbidities and impact of treatment choices.

Second

- Discuss plans and options with patient, family, and referring physician in the context of patient's goals.
- Anticipate and discuss benefits and burdens.
- Initiate preventative strategies to minimize likely burdens (e.g., drug-related side effects).

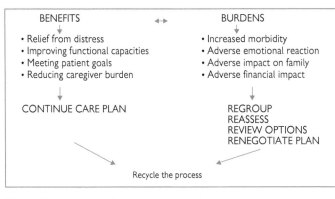

Figure 1.2 Assessing benefits and burdens

Third

- Monitor and assess impact of intervention.
- Weigh benefits versus burdens.

The Interdisciplinary Team (IDT)

The Functional Hospice IDT

While there are many elements that contribute to an exceptional hospice, the IDT is at its core. In fact, the interdisciplinary rather than multidisciplinary nature of hospice is what distinguishes it from conventional health care delivery structures. The more typical multidisciplinary group of health care professionals functions as several individuals with expertise in various areas working in serial fashion, separate from each other. Although overall objectives may be similar, they rarely work or meet together and even less frequently interact with the intent to overlap and interweave skill sets and care plans to arrive at those objectives. The multidisciplinary team is characterized by clear role definitions and consistent maintenance (even guarding) of the boundaries among those roles. A sports analogy would be a football or baseball team where each player has a specific position and assignment with only occasional deviation from these roles. Decision-making and authority are centralized by design, and there is little, if any, tolerance, let alone permission, for innovation.

The interdisciplinary group may be composed of identical professional members as the multidisciplinary paradigm, but the role definitions are purposefully blurred and the boundaries are widely overlapping. Authority is shared, as is decision-making, and innovation is encouraged wherever necessitated by patient need and circumstance. Referring to the previous sports analogy, the interdisciplinary group functions more like a basketball or soccer team where success results from fluid and spontaneous innovation, with some set plays but ample flexibility to adapt to the demands of changing situations. Roles are expected to be shared or traded as needed. In order to achieve this level of fluid teamwork, a high level of communication must be maintained, which requires considerable maturity, trust, and intimacy. These professional expectations may exceed those required in other, less-interdependent health care environments.

Such teams or groups require an unusual degree of attention to interpersonal relationships in order to maintain the necessary level of mutual trust and understanding of one another's strengths and limitations. This need exposes the team to a significant risk, however. In order to achieve and sustain the ideal level of professional intimacy, it is often necessary to engage in a level of sharing that feels more personal than professional to the team members. As a result, team members may begin to look to the team to meet their personal needs and even to resolve issues in their personal lives. This is the one boundary a team must not cross. To do so runs the risk of undermining the team's professional functioning and blurs the focus of the team: delivering the highest quality of care possible to patients in need.

To maintain an optimum functional level, team members often must share and explore emotional reactions their patients and families trigger in them. However, this sort of sharing and self-examination should always be undertaken to further their professional functions, not as a means of meeting personal needs. Those must be met outside of the work environment in the intimacy of one's own personal life or in one's own decisions to partake of professional help in sorting through difficult emotional experiences.

A high-functioning team must be flexible enough to reconfigure itself in response to the needs of each patient and family. This requires mature professionals who are able to deal with the personal and strong emotional issues hospice work engenders: one's own mortality, the motivations and sources that compel us to be a caretaker, one's need to be liked, ability to tolerate patients' anger, and so many others. While there can be intense and challenging issues, they should always and only be addressed in the effort to further the work at hand. We come together to assess and plan for the needs of our patients and families, not to address our own or our family's needs. The focus must always be the work: what serves the patient's and family's needs. The valuable time of team meetings needs to be spent addressing patient care issues first, then personal issues as necessary in order to fulfill the care plan, and finally interpersonal issues between or among team members when they become an impediment to care delivery. To depart from this healthy and functional approach is to depart from the reason the team exists.

The Structured Team Meeting

IDT Care Conference Format

This is a guide only, and it should be "molded" to fit the needs and unique circumstances of each team and the patients/families under care. Adherence to the *basic* format will ensure that most key issues are addressed and a focus on all pertinent elements is maintained. Keeping this format in mind during patient visits will also help to organize thinking and prioritize care issues.

Recommended IDT Conference Format for Patient Care Managers

- All disciplines represented and signed in
- Deaths reviewed since last IDT conference; lessons learned, thoughts and feelings about the care given and dying process

- New admissions (see "Two-minute" case presentation format below) in home and other residential care locations (nursing home, long-term care, assisted living) and inpatient settings
- Active problems (medical, psychosocial, practical, spiritual)
- Brief review of case load; indications for continuous care, inpatient admission (general inpatient and respite)
- Review patients who have been recertified since the last team meeting and review/schedule physician or nurse practitioner visits for those patients in need of a face-to-face visit (for recertification of hospice eligibility in benefit periods 3 and beyond) in the next 30 days; regulations regarding hospice recertification changed in January 2011, and may continue to do so; it is imperative that your Director of Compliance be involved in the interdisciplinary certification/recertification process so that your program is not vulnerable to loss of revenue due to technical denials
- A 15- to 20-minute mini "inservice" by team member(s) selected the previous week regarding a topic that emerged as "begging" deeper understanding and discussion by the team, or identified by patient care manager, such as symptom management, assessment/diagnosis, psychosocial issues, spiritual care issues, process/system (documentation, regulatory, compliance, etc.), bereavement
- Identification of topic and discussion leaders for next week's IDT conference "inservice"
- "Two-minute" case presentation by designated case manager, including patient name, age, gender, referring/primary physician, terminal diagnosis *(note: as much of this type of rostering that can be prepared in advance and automated, by using electronic media and projecting for the entire IDT to see, the better, because this will save time and reduce paper),* care situation (home, other); primary caregivers, current medications
  - Coexisting medical problems—Is there an adequate "database"? Is there a need for more information?
  - Interval history since last presentation
  - Symptoms well managed? Goals/needs met?
  - Continued problems, issues, needs, etc.
  - New problems, issues, needs, etc.
  - Progression of disease or level of debility (e.g., weight loss, decreased appetite, decreased energy/activity/function/ADLs, etc.); add specifics to documentation
- Review of determinants of limited prognosis for hospice admission diagnosis (supporting documents in medical record?)
- If symptoms are not well controlled, propose most likely etiology and specific treatment plan
- Communication with referring physician: when, how, what?
- Is communication profile on referring physician complete? (i.e., profile of type of communication [telephone call, fax, email, letter] by whom and how often preferred by referring/primary care physician)

- Focused discussion led by patient care manager with input from IDT on the five "quality of life" domains as they pertain to the ongoing care of the patient/family under review:
  - Physical symptoms (pain, nausea, etc.)
  - Physical functions (activity, etc.)
  - Intrapersonal dimension (emotional status, self-view, etc.)
  - Interpersonal status (relationships, communication, conflicts, etc.)
  - Transcendent issues (issues of "meaning," existence, spiritual matters, etc.)
- In relation to the major end outcomes of end-of-life care:
  - Safe and comfortable dying
  - Self-determined life closure
  - Effective coping with loss and grief
- The plan of care should be derived from the above, including plan for communication with referring physician, delegation of duties to specific IDT members (who, what, when, how often, goals), and next scheduled review by IDT

Addressing Needs Over Time

This section is meant as a guide for helping patients, families, and the caregiving team understand the dynamics of the last phase of life. Time frames represent generalizations that will need to be tailored to pertain to specific cases, but overall, they should help orchestrate care and prepare for the changes that tend to occur with advanced illness no matter where the patient resides.

Professional caregiver responsibilities, duties, and levels of involvement are assigned to those disciplines (core members of the IDT) that are most likely to have the greatest expertise in attending to the specified functions and needs of patients during the various phases of disease progression. These are not meant to be exclusive by any means. The true strength of the IDT is the ability of its core and additional members (e.g., pharmacists, nutritionists, functional restoration therapists), regardless of specific discipline, to fulfill multiple roles as the situation dictates, limited only by professional practice licensure restrictions and the experience and proven ability of the individual.

Hospice IDT Members: Approximately 6 Months or Longer Before Death

Patient and Family

- Patients are usually coherent and able to walk. They may have symptoms from previous medical treatments.
- Patient and family exhibit initial stages of grief with feelings of potential loss, anger, and denial.
- There may be humor and a heightened sense of living, all very appropriate.
- Some symptoms of decline (weight loss, fatigue) and a sense of the seriousness of the illness usually emerge.
- Initial signs of stress, with symptoms of depression, anxiety, or fear, should be anticipated and discussed.
- Family members wonder how they will cope.

Physician

- Reviews medical history; examines patient when indicated and certifies for hospice care
- Works with IDT to develop plan of care and authorizes medical orders
- Manages pain and other distressing symptoms
- Hospice physician attends interdisciplinary team meetings and confers with attending/referring physician as needed

RN/Case Manager

- Communicates with physician, family, and patient to develop initial plan of care
- Ensures that medical orders and durable medical equipment are in place and trains/instructs nonprofessional caregivers
- Coordinates plan of care, providing direct patient care and directs other nurses, aides, and volunteers
- Manages resources
- Establishes rapport and trust with patient, family, and attending physician
- Furthers discussions about advance care plans and end-of-life decisions
- Coordinates input at interdisciplinary team conferences

CNA/HHA

- Initiates personal care program under direction of RN case manager
- Establishes rapport with patient and family and provides personal care
- Conferences with case manager in developing care instructions

Social Worker

- Elaborates hospice philosophy and services
- Assesses patient and family needs from a psychosocial and spiritual perspective
- Collaborates in development of a plan of care according to needs, goals, preferences, and hopes
- Provides support, problem-solving, coping strategies, and connections to other community resources as needed

Chaplain

- Collaborates with other team members as care plan is developed
- Meets with patient and/or family at their request for spiritual or related care
- Helps other team members providing psychosocial support and dealing with difficult issues

Volunteer

- Volunteer manager collaborates with interdisciplinary team to determine patient/family needs that may be fulfilled by volunteers
- Arranges visits or telephone calls according to patient and family wishes and needs
- Assists with respite breaks and provides volunteer companionship when needed

Hospice IDT Members: A Few Months Before Death

Patient and Family

- Patient has decreased appetite, fatigue, and weight loss.
- Physical signs and symptoms are more evident. Family begins to reconcile feelings and plan for imminent death.
- Patient begins to accept the fact that disease is incurable and time is limited.
- Physical decline is apparent, and increased attention is spent on coping with progressive pain and other symptoms.
- Patient may show signs of social withdrawal, and the family may show signs of stress from caregiving and anticipatory grief.

Physician

- Works with IDT to evaluate symptoms, manage pain, and contribute to plan of care, adjusting medical orders as necessary
- Evaluates for continued hospice eligibility per guidelines

RN/Case Manager

- Monitors implementation of care plan with increasing attention to symptom management
- Assists IDT in evaluating and managing psychosocial needs

CNA/HHA

- Provides or assists in personal care as needed and directed
- Offers companionship
- Provides feedback to IDT about unmet needs and changes in status

Social Worker

- Monitors psychosocial plan of care and adapts it to changing needs and circumstances as they unfold
- Provides ongoing assessment of patient's and family's adjustment to the illness and impending loss and helps determine timing of respite based upon coping abilities
- Provides ongoing emotional support

Chaplain

- Provides spiritual and emotional support and counseling
- Communicates with clergy or lay spiritual leader of family/patient choosing
- Encourages and helps arrange rituals that offer meaning and support to the patient/family

Volunteer

- Works with volunteer coordinator, IDT, and patient/family to be aware of unspoken emotional or practical needs
- Spends "unstructured" time with patient and family in order to allow free exchange of concerns and feelings
- Helps relieve boredom for patient by engaging in whatever activities are feasible
- Works with IDT to identify ways and means to relieve caregiving burden

Hospice IDT Members: Last Few Weeks and Days

Patient and Family

- Symptoms tend to increase, with control of pain and shortness of breath chief symptom relief concerns.
- Fatigue becomes a dominant feature and the patient may be bedridden, requiring intensification of personal care and prevention of skin breakdown.
- The patient may alternately be extremely demanding and very withdrawn.
- Reinitiation of discussion regarding signs of imminent death, dealing with terminal care issues and funeral arrangements, is usually desired.

Physician

- Works with IDT to review symptoms with a focus on pain and other distressing symptom relief
- Contributes to biomedical aspects of the plan of care, adjusting medical orders as necessary
- Visits patient and family if symptoms are not readily controlled
- Available for rapid adjustment in medication orders and route of drug delivery as conditions dictate

RN/Case Manager

- Monitors patient closely, with increased frequency of home visits as dictated by changing conditions
- Frequent review of symptom control
- Coordinates care by members of IDT to support family and manage terminal care needs
- Determines whether continuous care or inpatient care is needed
- Instructs family in signs of imminent dying and to call so that attendance at death, or immediately thereafter, is possible

CNA/HHA

- Responds to changes in plan of care as directed by case manager
- Special attention to oral care, perineum, and pressure points
- Identifies special needs to IDT

Social Worker

- Anticipates and assesses for heightened anxiety and emotional distress, as well as caregiver fatigue
- Assists patient and family in resolving conflicts and making closure, expressing thoughts and feelings
- Helps family with funeral planning

Chaplain

- Continues to provide spiritual and emotional support
- Provides pastoral care as requested by the patient and family
- May assist with funeral arrangements and rituals

- Helps prepare family and patient for separation, and looks for ways to help heal relationships that are stressed, facilitating closure and the final opportunity for personal growth before death
- Familiarizes family with bereavement program, especially if bereavement counselor is a different person

Hospice IDT Members: After Death

- Family experiencing loss and grief

Physician

- May communicate with family; may send condolence note

RN/Case Manager

- Calls or visits family
- May attend funeral
- Assists bereavement counselor in assessing family's bereavement needs
- Completes documentation

CNA/HHA

- May attend funeral or visit family

Social Worker

- Calls or visits family
- May attend funeral
- Assesses family for signs of dysfunctional grieving and other psychosocial problems
- Makes referrals to appropriate resources

Chaplain/Bereavement

- May call or visit family
- May attend funeral
- Instructs family about grief recovery and support groups

Counselor

- Provides bereavement counseling as needed
- Plans and implements memorial services
- Directs staff and volunteers to maintain contact with family at regular intervals for 13 months

Volunteer

- May call or visit family
- May attend funeral
- Bereavement volunteers offer support for 13 months.

Documentation

The Clinical Documentation Process Serves Several Important Functions

- It is the structure that describes what is to be done, what has been done, and what has been accomplished to meet the patient's/family's goals.

- It is the continuous and memorialized record of the patient and his or her experiences through hospice.
- Well-constructed records provide unambiguous and clear communication among all hospice care staff.
- The medical record is the means by which reimbursement for services is justified and determined.

Documents Must Serve the Needs of Many Different Persons and Organizations

Patient/Family

- Informative documents, brief and to the point
- As few signatures as possible
- Confidentiality
- Pertinent information only (respect for privacy, dignity, ethical boundaries) for delivery of quality care

Attending Physician and Referral Sources

- Brief, complete, summarized information
- Minimal paperwork burden

Interdisciplinary Team and Administrative Personnel

- Legible and timely entries
- Access to information
- Complete information
- Logical flow of information

Clinical Facilities (e.g., hospital, nursing home, inpatient unit)

- Facilitate continuity of care
- Logical flow of plan of care
- Summary information, encapsulated to provide brief but complete picture of the patient and other pertinent facts at time of admission

Regulatory Agencies, Third-Party Payers, Accreditation Entities

- Proof of eligibility
- Zero tolerance for fraud/abuse of public funds
- Required for payment
- Critical step in regulatory compliance
- Complete entries
- Signed entries
- Adequate narrative to "tell the story" or "paint a picture" of the patient's/family's circumstances and experience through hospice
- Processes of care (evaluations, plans of care, interventions)
- Outcomes of care

Documentation and Risk Management

- Use full signature; date and time all entries.
- Complete all medical records and documentation forms (i.e., fill in the blanks).

- Be specific; elaborate only as necessary.
- Individual viewpoints are reviewed and reconciled at IDT conference, not in the written record. Discussions and challenge of ideas/perspectives are appropriate and welcome at IDT conference but have no place in the medical record.
- Report adverse occurrences/mistakes on incident reports.
- Legibility is key.
- Use only universally accepted abbreviations; when in doubt, spell it out.
- Read back verbal orders and note this confirmation to reduce medication errors.

Documentation Needs Specific to Hospice Care

- Routine home care: records must tell the story of the patient and reflect the patterns of care and the hospice experience.
- General inpatient care: records must clearly show the indications for a change in level of care.
  - Symptoms out of control
  - Efforts to regain control in the home
  - What interventions can be done in the inpatient setting that cannot be done at home?
  - Caregiver or environmental crisis needs to be well described
  - If death is imminent, describe findings in detail
  - Daily assessments, care plan, and IDT involvement need to be documented
  - All interventions must be charted in detail, taking nothing for granted
  - Specify what comfort measures were provided
  - Must have frequent documentation (i.e., every 1 to 2 hours), not a synopsis; no "block charting" (e.g., 1–4 a.m.); charting must include specific times and events
  - Document what the medical crisis was and continues to be that justifies this level of care
- Initial certification and recertification: supply ample narrative that describes clinical parameters with respect to the hospice diagnosis and ongoing trajectory toward death.
- Define as clearly as possible "related" and "unrelated" conditions and therapies in relation to hospice diagnosis (e.g., diuretics are related to the diagnosis of end-stage heart failure, whereas insulin would be unrelated to this diagnosis).
- Utilize prognostic worksheets and guidelines and supplement with observations that support a prognosis of limited life expectancy.
  - Track objective measures of decline (weight loss, reduced appetite, decreasing functional abilities, etc.)
  - When decline is not apparent, describe care that may be leading to functional improvement and plans to review prognosis if improvement in status is sustained

- Home health aide/certified nurse assistant supervisory visits: document supervision every 2 weeks—ensure compliance with state regulations.
- IDT communication: comprehensive care plan updates are essential
  - Summarize communications in easy-to-review form
  - Clearly state who (include discipline), what, when, why, anticipated goals, contingency plans, and next evaluation
- Nursing home documentation: the record must show an integrated plan of care that clearly and specifically delineates hospice functions and identifies responsible staff:
  - All care must be documented
  - Nursing home chart must have a specific place for hospice records
  - Medical orders must be duplicated and integrated into comprehensive plan of care

Accountability

- All hospice staff are individually responsible and accountable for completing their respective portion(s) of the medical record in a legible and timely manner—this is a fundamental expectation and there are no exceptions.
- The RN case manager is chiefly responsible and accountable for coordinating care and ensuring completeness of the medical records of the patients he or she is managing and, in turn, will monitor others' compliance. If deficiencies are not immediately corrected, the program director, or equivalent position, is to be notified so that corrective actions can be taken.

Section 2

Personal, Social, and Environmental Processes

Abuse in the Home

SITUATION: Domestic abuse or neglect interfering with end-of-life care

Findings

- Expression of ambivalent feelings of anger, jealousy, hurt, fear, sadness, guilt, self-righteousness, apologies, promises, or martyrdom
- Use of intimidation and manipulation as a way to maintain control and avoid feelings
- Family history of verbal, emotional, physical, economic, or sexual abuse
- Use of defense mechanisms: minimization, justification, denial, and blame
- Depression, suicidal ideation
- Physical evidence of abuse/neglect

Assessment

Physical

- Environmental or corporeal evidence of abuse, neglect, violence

Psychosocial

- Patient as victim of abuse
  - Identify patient/caregiver's perception of situation.
  - Assess history of abuse/neglect.
  - Assess patient fears.
  - Identify present threats of harm.
  - Identify if caregiver insists on staying close and speaking for patient.
  - Assess if patient is reluctant to speak or disagree in presence of caregiver.
  - Identify symptoms of depression, panic attacks, substance abuse, feelings of isolation, and post-traumatic stress reactions.
  - Determine patient/caregiver resources to address issue.
  - Determine support systems available.
  - Assess for risk of suicide.
- Patient as abuser
  - Identify patient/caregiver's perception of situation.
  - Assess safety if patient is still physically capable of abuse.

- Identify verbal and emotional abuse to caregiver by patient.
- Assess need for control, manipulation, intimidation.
- Assess presence of denial, minimization, justification, and blame as defense mechanisms.
- Identify caregiver's ambivalent feelings/desire for revenge as barrier to provide adequate patient care.
- Assess for intense emotional reaction to loss, including suicide potential.

Processes of Care

Psychosocial

- Patient as victim of abuse
  - Facilitate discussion of perceptions and feelings.
  - Acknowledge and encourage use of previously effective coping skills.
  - Assist patient/caregiver in accepting limits imposed by illness.
  - Assist patient/caregiver to develop new coping skills.
  - Provide education on safety issues.
  - See patient alone when possible.
  - Visit with two staff members, one to see caregiver and one to see patient, to obtain clear information.
  - Monitor willingness/ability to comply with treatment plan.
  - Consider transfer to alternative location (e.g., care facility) if need arises.
  - Confer with team members regarding intervention plan and options for care.
- Patient as abuser
  - Provide education on safety issues.
  - Develop safety plan with team and caregiver.
  - Assist in setting limits and clear communication about unacceptable behaviors with patient.
  - Encourage patient to identify feelings underneath anger and need for control.
  - Support caregiver in taking care of own needs.
  - Provide additional support to give caregiver respite.
  - Assist caregiver in making decisions on behalf of the patient that are not detrimental to caregiver.
  - Discuss alternative with caregiver in situations of high risk/burnout (e.g., care facility placement).
  - Confer with bereavement support staff regarding high risk for dysfunctional grief.

Goals/Outcomes

- Patient/caregiver will show improved ability to cope
- Patient/caregiver/hospice staff will be aware of need for clear limits/ boundaries for safety
- Patient/caregiver will identify strategies to address needs in the terminal situation
- Decreased incidence of domestic abuse/violence/neglect

Documentation in the Medical Record
Initial and Ongoing Physical Assessment
- Examination findings suggestive of abuse, neglect

Initial and Ongoing Psychosocial Assessment
- Areas of abuse, neglect, and violence as identified by patient, family, and staff

Interdisciplinary Progress Notes and IDT Care Plan
- Specific interventions to assist patient/caregiver
- Patient/caregiver response to intervention
- Ongoing evaluation

Advance Care Planning and Directives for Health-care Interventions

SITUATION: Patient has preferences about medical interventions and chooses to protect his/her rights by specifying the type of medical care desired.

State-specific advance directives can be obtained by accessing the NHPCO Caring Connections website via www.NHPCO.org

Findings
- Patient wants to make decisions and protect his/her rights
- Patient wants to clarify preferences to physician and caregiver/family
- Family has differing ideas about treatment for patient
- Patient wants to communicate choices while still able

Assessment
Psychosocial
- Assess if advance directives have been previously completed
- Assess patient/caregiver's awareness/understanding of value/purpose of advance directives
- Assess patient's desire to complete forms with or without assistance from hospice staff

Processes of Care
Psychosocial
Educate patient and family about different types of advance directives and processes:
- Power of Attorney

Patient gives power to transact business on his/her behalf when he/she cannot do so because of time or distance (although physically able).
- Durable Power of Attorney

Patient gives power to transact business on his/her behalf when patient is no longer physically able.
- Living Will

This is an advance directive that states what types of care or medical interventions patient prefers or wishes to avoid under various circumstances.

- Durable Power of Attorney for Health Care

This legal document protects patient care choices by naming an advocate who makes decisions on behalf of patient when physician determines patient is not competent.

- Do Not (Attempt to) Resuscitate

This directive states that the patient refuses certain *potentially* life-prolonging medical interventions, such as cardiopulmonary resuscitation, chest compressions, endotracheal intubation, and defibrillation.

- Physician Orders for Life-Sustaining Treatment (POLST)

Forms and educational programs intended to facilitate the greatest amount of patient self-determination in making end-of-life treatment decisions. This paradigm varies by state, with educational tools and forms for consumers and healthcare professionals. More information can be obtained by accessing the website www.ohsu.edu/polst/ (accessed December, 2011).

Guardianship

Parent is the guardian for minor child unless a legal action rules otherwise. Court-appointed guardianship by petition can be temporary, financial, or custodial.

- Facilitate discussion regarding choices for treatment/care with family when patient is no longer able to participate in these decisions.
- Facilitate discussion with patient/caregiver regarding appropriate advance directives and choice of advocate.
- Assist patient in completing advance directives form/document.
- Procure a copy of advance directive for patient record.

Goals/Outcomes

- Patient will voice preferences about current and future medical care and actions to be taken in the event of loss of decision-making ability
- Caregiver/family/advocate will have clear directions for understanding patient choices
- Minimize ambiguity and ambivalence in all parties
- Completion of life in a manner and setting consistent with wishes and values (i.e., "self-determined life closure"

Documentation in the Medical Record

Initial Psychosocial Assessment

- Need for advance directives as identified by patient/caregiver/social work/ admission team
- Options discussed
- Forms/documents completed
- Copy of advance directives and documents in medical record

Interdisciplinary Progress Notes
- Documentation of processes of advance care planning that have been completed

IDT Care Plan
- Plan for carrying out processes of advance care planning

Changes in Body Image and Loss of Independence

SITUATION: Patient/caregiver reactions to changes in body image and loss of independence associated with advanced illness causing distress and difficulty coping/functioning

Findings
- Persistent, preoccupying, and intense expressions of anger, frustration, lone-liness, loss of self-esteem, embarrassment, shame, guilt, etc. due to altered physical appearance, altered functional ability, changes in social/family identity/status
- Avoidance of discussion regarding appearance
- Loss of functional abilities due to disease process
- Increasing dependence upon others for care
- Caregiver loss of previously relied upon companion support; change in roles
- Social isolation
- Self-imposed disengagement from feelings, family members, friends, outside community
- Pronounced depression
- Sexual dysfunction
- Suicidal thoughts

Assessment
Physical
- Identify disease-related, postsurgical, or postradiation alterations in external physical features or means to communicate (e.g., amputation [including mas-tectomy; orchiectomy]; ostomies; open sores/wounds/lesions; scars or other disfigurement; vocal/visual/auditory impairment)

Psychosocial/Spiritual
- Identify primary issue(s) of concern
- Explore patient/caregiver perception of body image, value of appearance, functional limitations
- Determine patient/caregiver capacity to address the issues
- Determine support systems available and nature/basis of faith/beliefs
- Identify who patient will allow to help provide care
- Assess for history of suicidal ideation or behavior
- Rule out other confounding issues/comorbidities (e.g., depression, anxiety disorder, agoraphobia)

- Identify history/style of coping
- Assess impact of illness/appearance upon sexuality
- Assess financial resources available for supplementary help if needed

Processes of Care

Physical

- Ensure that expert-level attention to wound and ostomy care, prosthetics, and other restorative or rehabilitative therapies, appropriate to the patient's overall circumstances, is arranged

Psychosocial/Spiritual

- Facilitate expressions of feelings and perceptions; acknowledge losses
- Address real versus perceived body image and functional limitations
- Acknowledge and encourage use of previously effective coping skills
- Provide information regarding progression of illness
- Assist patient/caregiver to develop new coping skills for positive self-image
- Encourage patient/caregiver participation in support groups
- Treat identified mood disorder/phobic behavior with counseling
- If symptoms are not responding to basic counseling approaches, assist in providing resources/referral to treat mood disorder/phobic behavior and support patient/family through crisis periods
- Assist patient in finding meaning in past achievements through life review

Practical

- Obtain consultation or access resources for use of prostheses, wigs, cosmetics, etc.
- Facilitate placement for respite and/or residential care if needed

Biomedical

- Treat identified mood disorder with pharmacotherapy if indicated, per severity and diagnostic criteria

Goals/Outcomes

- Condition-specific optimum physical and communicative capacities
- Patient/caregiver will demonstrate or verbalize improved coping ability
- Patient/caregiver will express higher level of acceptance of alterations in body image and changes in functional abilities
- Patient will exhibit less signs/symptoms of depression, anxiety, phobic behavior
- Patient will feel less isolated

Documentation in the Medical Record

Initial and Ongoing Physical Assessment

- Relevant physical findings and changes over time

Initial Psychosocial Assessment

- Evidence of poor body image/dependency and inadequate coping

Interdisciplinary Progress Notes
- Manifestations of changes in body image and loss of independence
- Ongoing assessments and results of interventions

IDT Care Plan
- Defined interventions and expected outcomes

Changes in Family Dynamics

SITUATION: Family dynamics are having a negative impact upon effective end-of-life care

Findings
- Family member(s) report high level of stress due to inability to cope effectively with crisis of impending death and eventual loss of patient
- Family member(s) exhibit difficulty with intimacy (dependency, conflict, or detachment)
- Family member(s) express concern/confusion about changes in roles, duties, lifestyle, and family interaction patterns
- Family member(s) report other existing stressful issues requiring time and attention

Assessment
Psychosocial/Spiritual
- Outline a "family tree" that describes the family system and defines roles, expectations, relationships, and issues
- Identify family interaction patterns (e.g., close, conflicted, enmeshed, distant, or estranged)
- Ask family member(s) to describe their perception of family in the context of the patient's terminal illness
- Identify previous experiences and patterns of dealing with loss individually and as a family system
- Assess appearance of harmony or disharmony among various family members
- Assess impact of conflicts on care of patient
- Assess position the patient maintains within the family structure
- Assess ability of family to communicate about dying
- Assess existence of self-destructive/family-impacting behaviors (e.g., substance abuse, gambling or other addictive disorders) with any immediate family members, including the patient
- Assess history of mental illness, abuse, or antisocial behavior
- Assess factors of illiteracy, or mental and physical limitations
- Assess experiences and attitudes of family in dealing with the medical community or with authority figures

- Assess willingness and ability to understand and utilize instructions and interventions
- Assess impact of ethnic/cultural background, values, beliefs, attitudes, and family rituals/traditions
- Assess ability of family system to access internal and external resources

Processes of Care

Psychosocial/Spiritual

- Facilitate discussion of useful strengths and resources that helped family member(s) in previous crises (e.g., cohesion, concern for each other, commitment to family, pride, loyalty, utilization of external resources)
- Increase awareness of family rules, boundaries, patterns of communication, and role expectations
- Encourage dialogue and expressions of feelings about illness and dying, when appropriate
- Identify role-change strain/conflict and assist in redistribution of roles and responsibilities
- Assist family member(s) in setting short-, intermediate-, and long-term goals and acknowledge progress made in achieving them
- Facilitate discussion of previous or ongoing hurt feelings that have potential for resolution/healing
- Facilitate referral to external resources as needed
- Facilitate arrangements for respite care, if appropriate, in family with high level of stress
- Assist family in shared life review and reminiscence, if appropriate
- Assist family in the task of preparing for the death of a family member
- Assist family in the task of beginning to prepare for life after the death of the family member
- Assist family in having realistic expectations of hospice care
- Provide emotional support to family
- Deal with resistance to psychosocial interventions
- Develop plan of care with patient, family, and interdisciplinary team and continue to monitor progress
- Facilitate family conference

Goals/Outcomes

- Family shows increased ability to cope with the imminent death of a family member in the context of the family system
- Family feels reduction in levels of stress
- Family will have strengthened external/internal resources to care for patient at home, if this is the most appropriate setting

Documentation in the Medical Record

Initial Psychosocial/Spiritual Assessment

- Dynamics of family system affecting care of terminally ill patient

Interdisciplinary Progress Notes
- Summary of IDT conferences related to family dynamics affecting care
- Results of interventions
- Summary of ongoing evaluations

IDT Care Plan
- Resources and problem-solving skills to be relayed/taught/recommended
- Social work interventions: who, what, when, how often; and specify goals
- Chaplain interventions: who, what, when, how often; and specify goals

Completing Worldly Business and Life Closure

SITUATION: Patient has a need to complete certain
tasks before death.

Findings
- Patient expressing lack of completion in worldly affairs
- Patient/caregiver expressing desire for completion with relationships
- Patient expressing "weariness" with life; lack of purpose/meaning in living
- Patient/caregiver unable to accept patient's death
- Patient/caregiver unable to resolve spiritual issues
- Patient/caregiver working toward balance of body, mind, and spirit in the face of death

Assessment
Psychosocial/Spiritual
- Identify patient/caregiver perception of situation
- Identify patient/caregiver capacity to address life closure and/or unresolved issues
- Review past life experiences, changes in roles, losses, and previously effective coping skills
- Identify role-change strain/conflict
- Identify patient/caregiver experiences, concerns, and fears regarding the dying process
- Assess need for spiritual care and anticipatory grief support
- Assess patient/caregiver perception of current quality of life and future concerns

Processes of Care
Psychosocial/Spiritual—Worldly Affairs
- Support patient/caregiver in settling financial affairs and making final arrangements
- Link patient/caregiver with appropriate resources: financial/estate planner, viatical settlement organizations, legal counsel, etc.
- Facilitate patient's writing of an estate will

Psychosocial/Spiritual—Meaning and Purpose in Life

- Assist patient in coming to terms with personal and existential loss represented by one's dying
- Facilitate patient/caregiver expressed need to search for meaning in the dying experience
- Review past life experiences, role changes, and losses
- Reinforce previously effective coping skills
- Help patient/caregiver search the meaning and depth of his or her particular faith/beliefs
- Assist patient in acceptance of dependence
- Refer to "complementary" therapies: music, art, massage, etc.
- Assist patient toward growth/development in the context of personal grieving, loss, and suffering
- Relationships
  - Present grief as a unique opportunity to address and heal unresolved issues and fears.
  - Facilitate closure with important relationships by expressing sorrow, forgiveness, affection, love, gratitude, appreciation, and saying "goodbye."
  - Assist patient in expressing self-worth and forgiveness.
  - Involve caregiver in planning for emotional, spiritual, psychosocial, and physical needs and facilitate implementation.
  - Facilitate discussion of useful strengths and resources that helped family members in previous crises.
  - Identify role-change strain/conflict and assist in redistribution of roles/responsibilities.
  - Assist family in the task of preparing for the death of the patient.
  - Facilitate and validate family rituals.
  - Assist family in the task of beginning to prepare for life after the death of the patient.
  - Refer, as appropriate, to grief support counselor for anticipatory grief.

Psychosocial/Spiritual—Dying

- Respond to questions and concerns about the signs and symptoms indicating patient is approaching death
- Explore patient/caregiver experiences, concerns, and fears regarding dying process
- Support patient in letting go of worldly affairs and surrendering to the transcendent

Spiritual Issues

- Explore issues of guilt and human and/or divine forgiveness
- Encourage spiritual practices of meditation, keeping a written journal or audio/visual tape, imagery, prayers, and/or spiritual/religious rites
- Explore belief, faith, and trust in higher dimension that provide patient/caregiver support

- Assess need for spiritual care
- Respond to specific pastoral requests
- Encourage emotional/spiritual sharing among patient/family members
- Facilitate patient/caregiver connection with his or her preferred religious institution, if any

Goals/Outcomes

- Patient/caregiver will express increased sense of completion in worldly affairs
- Patient/caregiver will express increased sense of meaning and purpose
- Patient/caregiver will express increased sense of completion with relationships
- Patient/caregiver is able to express acceptance of his/her death if possible
- Patient/caregiver will feel that there has been resolution of spiritual issues
- Patient/caregiver will have a sense of personal completion to life

Documentation in the Medical Record

Initial Psychosocial/Spiritual Assessment

- Major emotional, psychosocial, and spiritual issues of concern identified by patient, family, and hospice staff
- Coping skills, resources, preferences identified

Interdisciplinary Progress Note

- Continued identification of issues as per initial assessment
- Ongoing identification of goals
- Results and goals/outcomes summarized

IDT Care Plan

- Interventions planned by staff (who, what, when, frequency, goals)
- Plans for ongoing evaluation

Controlled Substances: Misuse and Abuse

SITUATION: Medically inappropriate use of controlled substances in the home having a negative impact on end-of-life care

Findings

- Pattern of unexplained disappearance of medications
- Consistent shortage of prescribed controlled substance without appropriate communication to care team about medical necessity to change dose or schedule
- History or evidence of substance use among patient, family, and friends
- Deliberate guarding or expression of need to guard medications from others
- Environmental clues that suggest drug diversion
- Unusual patient or family perceptions of symptom management

Assessment

Psychosocial/Spiritual

- Identify substance abuse as reported by patient/caregiver and/or observed by professional care team member(s)
- Identify characteristics of chemically dependent family system as evidenced by the following patterns:
  - Denial
  - Control
  - Conflict
  - Distrust
  - Unresolved losses
  - Secrets
  - Resistance to outsiders
  - Blaming
  - Domestic chaos
  - Violence
  - Falsification
- Identify prior or current use of formal treatment and support programs (i.e., AA, NA, ALANON, NARANON, etc.)
- Understand patient and family perceptions regarding symptom management and substance abuse
- Assess impact of substance use on ability to provide patient care or to cope with dying
- Refer to the *Diagnostic & Statistical Manual, Fourth Edition (DSM-IV-TR)* in completing assessment
- Assess need to intervene and/or refer to specialty counseling or mental health services based on impact of substance abuse
- Understand special social/cultural/ethnic/religious perspectives (rituals) of patient/caregiver/family member(s) on controlled substance use

Processes of Care

Educational

- Provide information regarding effects of substance abuse on physical symptoms and grief processes
- Provide information and instruction regarding achievable expectations regarding symptom management

Psychosocial/Spiritual

- Explore motivations for substance use (abuse), especially if a new problem
  - Depression/despair/hopelessness
  - Anxiety
  - Fear
  - Anticipated grief
  - Other conflicts
- Involve family in talking about options and interventions
- Use appropriate referral sources
- Develop unified team approach

Practical/Procedural

- Schedule II/III medicines (e.g., opioids, benzodiazepines) are to be reordered by only one nurse
- Renew only 1-week supply at a time
- Count medication carefully each nursing visit

Goals/Outcomes

- Patient/caregiver will verbalize understanding of appropriate medical use of prescription medications for symptom management (schedule and dose)
- Patient/family will utilize outside resources for specific issues related to substance abuse as necessary to attain patient end-of-life goals
- Effect(s) of substance abuse on patient care or ability to cope will be minimized

Documentation in the Medical Record

Initial Psychosocial/Spiritual Assessment

- Explicit findings of substance abuse
- Current and projected impact on patient/caregiver/family

Interdisciplinary Progress Note

- Interventions carried out (who, what, when)
- Expected goals/outcomes
- Results of interventions
- Findings of ongoing evaluations and assessments

IDT Care Plan

- Schedule of interventions
- Contingency plans if interventions do not achieve hoped-for outcomes
- Schedule of follow-up and reevaluations
- Changes in care plan with justification

Cultural Differences: Respect, Understanding, and Adapting Care

Note: The citizenry of the United States is ethnically, religiously, and racially diverse. This brief overview is meant to serve as both a reminder and a guide so that professional caregivers can meet the varied needs of individuals within our culturally heterogeneous society.

SITUATION: The patient/family under care has significantly different values and customs than the professional caregivers.

Findings: Initial and ongoing patient/family assessment will reveal a wide range of cultural differences, such as

- Country of origin, sense of nationality, ethnic background
- Language, dress, interpersonal behavior and interpretation of caregivers' spoken and "body" language (e.g., eye contact, "personal space," manners/mannerisms, etc.)
- Attitudes toward individuality, autonomy, self-determination, and place within the family and society

- Attitudes toward illness, dependency, dying, and death
- Attitudes toward food, meals, and nutrition
- Attitudes toward pain and suffering
- Attitudes toward modesty and gender roles
- Expression of spirituality: religion/religious institution, faith, rituals, beliefs

Assessment, Processes of Care, Goals/Outcomes, Documentation

In order to provide meaningful end-of-life care, a thorough understanding of the patient's/family's cultural imperatives and values is necessary. This may be particularly challenging when there are language barriers, so every reasonable attempt should be made to obtain capable translation. If at all possible, caregivers or volunteers should be assigned who have some experience with the particular cultural values system of the patient/family, and the IDT can then be better educated to the particular nuances that will affect care.

The entire hospice team needs to be committed to providing assistance without prejudice to all people with limited life expectancy who want our help. This mission demands the highest regard for individual rights and freedoms in accordance with the laws of the land. Due to the diversity of people in our society, it is more likely than not that we will encounter individuals who are very different from ourselves. In order to be true to the principle of patient-centered and family-focused care, insight into the values of those who invite us into this phase of their lives is a necessity. Only through conscious attempts at understanding can unintended bias and unwitting "cultural blunders" be prevented.

It is beyond the scope of this manual to elaborate all the various cultural differences that exist toward dying and death. Nevertheless, the hospice professional is encouraged to expand his or her knowledge with an open-minded and inquisitive attitude whenever the opportunity presents itself. There are many resources for learning in every community: church groups, cultural organizations, local libraries, and the Internet, among other sources, can provide helpful background. And, under most circumstances, patients and families are extremely pleased that someone is interested in seeing the world through their eyes. Most important, your willingness to understand and appreciate others' life views in the midst of their coming to terms with life and death will be valued beyond measure.

Denial

SITUATION: Problematic expressions of denial that interfere with attainment of patient-directed goals, care of patient, ability to cope

Findings

- Family insists that patient not be told prognosis
- Resistance to accepting available support and help to the extent that inadequate care is rendered and patient goals are not able to be realistically assessed/attained
- Preoccupation with somatic symptoms with a view toward rediagnosis/cure in the face of appropriate diagnostic/prognostic information given
- Inability to acknowledge patient's physical and/or mental decline

- Excessive resistance to planning for future without patient
- Excessive resistance to talk about prognosis
- Patient/family making unrealistic future plans

Assessment
Psychosocial/Spiritual

- Explore and understand patient and caregiver's perception of situation
- Explore and understand motivations for (purposes served by) denial
- Assess history of coping style with prior losses
- Assess impact of denial on family dynamics, symptom management, safety issues, and ability to cope
- Review and understand beliefs/faith and support systems of patient/caregiver/family

Processes of Care
Practical

- Educate caregiver/family and care team about denial as a usual and healthy coping strategy, and the potential for maladaptive denial to interfere with good care and the attainment of goals

Psychosocial/Spiritual

- Approach denial openly, thoroughly supporting it as a constructive self-protective coping mechanism
- As appropriate, assist patient, caregiver, and family to confront the issues of denial and develop plans to achieve relief of unresolved concerns
- Assist patient/caregiver to develop alternate constructive coping strategies as situation dictates

Goals/Outcomes

- Patient/caregiver will address denial as barrier to patient care
- Maladaptive coping styles will decrease, at least to the extent that adequate assessment of realistic and potentially attainable goals and care can take place
- Patient/caregiver will more productively understand/utilize denial as an adjustment mechanism and as a response to loss to enhance remaining time before death
- Patient/caregiver will make progress toward making final plans and funeral arrangements

Documentation in the Medical Record
Initial Psychosocial/Spiritual Assessment

- Degree to which denial is playing a role in coping
- Evidence of maladaptive denial: interference with ability to adequately evaluate goals, expectations, hopes, etc.; interference with ability to ensure basic safety and/or quality care
- Risk for lack of closure and/or pathological grief

Interdisciplinary Progress Note

- Ongoing area(s) of denial
- Interventions and outcomes

IDT Care Plan

- Schedule of interventions: who, what, when
- Contingency plans if first set of approaches not beneficial
- Schedule of follow-up and reevaluation: who, when

Grief Reactions

SITUATION: Excessive grief interfering with patient/caregiver ability to function or cope

Findings

- Excessive sadness, anger, guilt, anxiety, loneliness, fatigue, hopelessness, numbness (lack of attachment, dissociation), helplessness
- Sleep disturbance
- Eating disturbance
- Social withdrawal
- Restless or frenetic activity/compulsive or repetitive behaviors
- Somatic preoccupation, symptoms
- Mood disturbance (depression, mania)
- Impulsive behaviors
- Functional impairment
- Suicidal ideation
- Onset or exacerbation of addictive behaviors, including eating, smoking, alcohol abuse, gambling

Assessment

Psychosocial/Spiritual

- Identify cultural background, traditions, and attitudes regarding death/grief
- Understand spiritual beliefs/religious affiliation and practices
- Understand how family expresses emotions
- Define realistic parameters of life expectancy/prognosis
- Determine the patient's role in the family and the potential impact of the loss
- Review prior history of previous experiences with loss and coping style/skills
- Assess suicide potential/ideation
- Assess support systems
- Assess substance abuse, if indicated

Biomedical

- Evaluate sleep patterns, eating patterns, mood, functional limitations, suicide risk

Interdisciplinary Team

- IDT to review, compare, and consolidate findings in order to determine the degree to which anticipatory grief is maladaptive and harmful

Processes of Care

Psychosocial/Spiritual

- Provide information on the grieving process
- Encourage patient/caregiver to talk about his/her losses

- Involve family in problem-solving/goal-setting
- Assist patient/caregiver to identify and express emotions
- Reinforce positive coping strategies
- Suggest and help develop new or more adaptive coping strategies
- Reinforce benefit of caregiver involvement in directly caring for patient and acknowledge/validate these efforts
- Encourage participation in physical and social activities
- Encourage expressive activities such as writing, painting, music, crafts, gardening, etc.
- Elicit preferences and facilitate family rituals
- Mobilize bereavement support resources, including extended family, friends, community groups, religious organization or other spiritual care when valued by patient/caregiver/family
- Facilitate funeral planning with patient/caregiver
- Slowly and carefully assist caregiver to explore ways to restructure life without patient
- Identify complicated and pathological grief reactions and refer to appropriate mental health resource
- Encourage participation in grief support programs
- Consult with bereavement support staff

Biomedical
- Treat disordered mood and sleep with appropriate medications on a short-term basis if not rapidly responsive to nonpharmacological approaches

Goals/Outcomes

- Patient/caregiver will verbalize understanding of normal grief response
- Caregiver will utilize grief support services as appropriate
- Patient/caregiver will express emotions related to grief
- Patient/caregiver will verbalize sense of increased ability to cope with grief
- Extreme and pathological grief reactions will be identified early so that appropriate resources can be mobilized

Documentation in the Medical Record
Initial Psychosocial/Spiritual Assessment
- Grief reactions manifested by patient/caregiver

Interdisciplinary Progress Note
- Ongoing observations and evaluation of grief reactions
- Results of specific interventions

IDT Care Plan
- Specific interventions: who, what, when, how often
- Contingencies for poor response to primary interventions

NOTE: Processes of grief and bereavement in children depend on developmental age (Table 2.1). Anticipated and aberrant reactions must be readily distinguished and specially trained (pediatric) staff must intercede quickly when unhealthy behaviors are evident.

Table 2.1 Grief and Bereavement in Children

Characteristics of Age	View of Death and Response	What Helps
BIRTH TO SIX MONTHS		
• Basic needs must be met, cries if needs are not met	• Has no concept of death	• Progressively disengage child from primary caregiver if possible.
• Needs emotional and physical closeness of a consistent caregiver	• Experiences death like any other separation—no sense of "finality"	• Introduce a new primary caregiver.
• Derives identity from caregiver	• Nonspecific expressions of distress (crying)	• Nurturing, comforting
• View of caregiver as source of comfort and all needs fulfillment	• Reacts to loss of caregiver	• Anticipate physical and emotional needs and provide them.
	• Reacts to caregiver's distress	• Maintain routines.
SIX MONTHS TO TWO YEARS		
• Begins to individuate	• May see death as reversible	• Needs continual support, comfort
• Remembers face of others, caregiver when absent	• Experiences bona fide grief	• Avoid separation from close physical and emotional connections.
• Demonstrates full range of emotions, feelings, and interactions	• Grief response only to death of significant person in child's life	• Support caregiver to reduce distress and maintain a stable environment.
• Identifies caregiver as source of good	• Maintain daily structure and schedule	• Acknowledge sadness that loved one will not return—offer comfort.
• No control over feelings and responses; anticipate regressive behavior	• Screams, panics, withdraws, becomes disinterested in food, toys, activities	
	• Reacts in concert with distress experienced by caregiver	
TWO YEARS TO FIVE YEARS		
• Egocentric	• Sees death like sleep: reversible	• Remind him or her that loved one will not return.
• Cause–effect not understood	• Believes in magical causes	• Give realistic information, answer questions.
• Developing conscience	• Has sense of loss	• Involve in "farewell" ceremonies.

- Developing trust
- Attributes life to objects
- Feelings expressed mostly by behaviors
- Can recall events from past

| | - Help put words to feelings; provide ways to remember loved one. |
| - Keep home environment structured, stable. |
| - Encourage questions, expression of feelings. |
| - Reassure child who will take care of him or her. |

FIVE TO NINE YEARS

- Attributes life to things that move; may fear the dark.
- Begins to develop intellect
- Begins to relate cause and effect; understands consequences
- Literal, concrete, may feel responsible
- Decreasing fantasy life, increasing control of feelings

- Curiosity, questioning
- Anticipate regression, clinging
- Aggressive behavior common
- Worries about who will care for him or her

- Personifies death as ghosts, "bogeyman"
- Interest in biological aspects of life and death
- Begins to see death as irreversible
- May see death as punishment; needs strong parent
- Problems concentrating on tasks; may deny or hide feelings, vulnerability

- Give clear and realistic information.
- Include child in funeral ceremonies if he or she chooses.
- Give permission to express feelings and provide opportunities; reduce guilt by providing factual information.
- Maintain structured schedule, individual and family activities.
- Notify school of what is occurring, gentle confirmation, reassurance.

PREADOLESCENT THROUGH TEENS

- Individuation outside home
- Identifies with peer group; needs family attachment
- Understands life processes; can verbalize feelings
- Physical maturation

- Views death as permanent
- Sense of own mortality; sense of the future
- Strong emotional reactions; may regress, revert to fantasy
- May somaticize, intellectualize, morbid preoccupation

- Unambiguous information
- Provide opportunities to express self, feelings; encourage outside relationships with mentors.
- Provide tangible means to remember loved one; encourage self-expression, verbal and nonverbal.
- Dispel fears about physical concerns; educate about maturation; provide outlets for energy and strong feelings (recreation, sports, etc.); needs mentoring and direction.

Living Environment, Finances, and Support Systems

SITUATION: Inadequacy of living environment, finances, or support systems that interferes with patient care or ability of patient/caregiver to cope with illness/dying

Findings

- No caregiver or frail or otherwise limited caregiver
- Insufficient food, heat, electrical power, protection from extremes of weather
- Infestation
- Hazards (e.g., faulty wiring, heating, waste disposal/sanitation, or structures; unsecured weapons [guns, rifles, ammunition])
- Dangerous behaviors (e.g., smoking with oxygen or unattended while in bed)
- Isolation (e.g., inadequate transportation/telephone or inability to communicate due to language barrier or other communication problem)
- Insufficient financial resources for basic needs or expenses associated with illness and dying
- Ongoing or imminent legal matters, disputes

Assessment

Psychosocial/Practical

- Assess physical environment, and understand social support systems and extent of resources
- Identify legal decision-makers for patient
- Understand needs and wants of patient/caregiver; desire to change
- Define barriers to improving compromised situation
- Define financial and practical needs: food, shelter, heating/cooling, phone, transportation, funeral and burial expenses, uncovered medical expenses, legal expenses
- Determine unrealized sources of federal, state, and community assistance
- Help to determine current and future expense, income, and assets

Processes of Care

Psychosocial/Practical

- Address environmental concerns with patient/caregiver
- Develop action plan among team to help make environmental improvements as acceptable to patient (utilize volunteers and community resource networks)
- Provide home safety education and plan
- If safety and other basic concerns cannot be corrected, facilitate placement in a more secure environment if acceptable
- Determine extent to which patient/caregiver will accept volunteers, home health aide, continuous care, and respite care to provide needed support

- Provide information and help to procure financial assistance and social services, assist with application processes, and serve as liaison/facilitator/advocate with institutions and agencies
- Offer help with budgeting

Basic Home Safety

Environment

- Electrical safety: risk of electrical shock or fire
  - Remove electrical cords from beneath carpet and rugs.
  - Recommend replacement of worn, cracked, spliced, frayed electrical cords.
  - Reduce extension cord and multiple outlet adaptor overload.
- Floor safety: risk of falls and injury
  - Remove or secure loose rugs, runners, mats with appropriate fixation (tacks, adhesives, rubberized matting).
  - Secure loose carpet edges.
  - Recommend repair of uneven walkways or damaged flooring.
- Outside communication: help in case of emergency
  - If at all possible, place telephone where it is most accessible most of the time.
  - Emergency telephone numbers should be posted on or near telephone in large bold print.
- Fire safety
  - Recommend one smoke detector on every level of home.
  - Develop evacuation plan or review existing one with patient/caregiver; assign specific roles to capable live-in family members in case of fire.
  - Establish clear pathways to all exits.
  - Have key(s) accessible near key-locked (deadbolt) doors.
  - Inquire if actively used chimneys have been inspected; recommend annual inspection.
  - Kerosene heaters, wood stoves, and fireplaces should not be left unattended while in use.
- Bathroom safety
  - Tubs and showers should have nonskid surface/mats to prevent slips and falls.
  - Grab bars to assist transfers should be installed in tub, shower, and toilet area as needed.
  - Adjust hot water heater temperature to avoid burns; check water temperature on sensitive body part before bathing/showering (patients with sensory neuropathy are particularly vulnerable).
  - Use nightlights in the bathroom and hallways en route to bathroom.

- Bed safety
  - Assess need for pressure sore prevention and bed rails, and obtain safe/ effective equipment as indicated.
- Stairs and passageway safety
  - Stairs, hallways, and passageways between rooms should be well lit and free of clutter.
  - Stairs should have sturdy, well-secured handrails on both sides.
  - Avoid using stairs while wearing only socks or smooth-soled shoes/ slippers.
- Outdoors
  - Entrance ways should be clear of leaves, snow, and ice.
  - Recommend and assist with making arrangements to clear entryways in snowy weather.

Medical Supplies

General

- Storage: keep supplies in a cool, dry, clean area protected from children and pets
- Handling: make sure patient/caregiver has been given proper instruction on use and handling of all medical supplies and equipment, especially avoidance of injury and contamination
- Disposal: instruct patient/caregiver that all dressing materials and disposable equipment that has been in patient contact should be wrapped in newspaper, bagged, and placed in a completely secure trash area

Oxygen

- Storage: oxygen and tubing should be kept away from open flames or heat sources
- Handling: should be handled only by people who have been properly instructed by nursing personnel or medical equipment representatives
- Disposal: used tubing should be disposed of in the manner described above; all other equipment should be removed only by professional personnel

Drugs

- Storage: cool, dry place, secure from children and pets
  - Determine the best balance between safety and convenience for the patient/caregiver.
  - Determine whether medications require special handling or refrigeration. Review expiration dates.
- Handling: ensure that all medications are adequately labeled
  - Check name, dose, and time schedule before giving/taking any medication.
  - Observe patient taking medications to determine independent capability.
  - Give instruction for refilling prescriptions on a schedule prior to using up current medication supply.
  - Count medication doses on a regular basis for those prescriptions to be taken on an "around the clock" schedule to ensure appropriate utilization.

- Disposal: old, unused, or discontinued controlled substances should be flushed down the toilet; for a complete list of drugs that should be flushed, refer to:
- http://www.fda.gov/Drugs/ResourcesForYou/Consumers/BuyingUsing MedicineSafely/EnsuringSafeUseofMedicine/SafeDisposalofMedicines/ ucm186187.htm#MEDICINES (accessed December, 2011)
    - Chemotherapy drugs must be returned to the hospital for disposal.
    - When in doubt, speak to pharmacist.

Needles and Syringes ("Sharps")
- Storage: cool, dry place, secure from children and pets
- Handling: examine for signs of contamination before opening
    - All caregivers and patient need to be instructed in proper use, protection, and disposal.
    - Observe caregiver/patient capability prior to independent use.
- Disposal: place used "sharps" in supplied puncture-resistant container to be returned to the hospice office for disposal

Infectious Waste
- Storage: do not store
- Handling: use gloves, confine to patient area, secure all materials in double plastic bags
- Disposal: flush all excretions/secretions down the toilet
    - Dispose of contaminated materials as described above.
    - Cleanse reusable containers by soaking in a 1:10 dilution of household bleach for at least 30 minutes.

Parenteral and Enteral Solutions
- Storage
    - Store unopened enteral solutions/mixes at room temperature and administer at room temperature.
    - Opened cans or mixes for enteral feeding must be covered, dated and timed, and refrigerated and should be used within 24 hours of opening.
    - Parenteral solutions should be stored in a refrigerator (except lipids) and removed 1 hour prior to administration.
    - Parenteral solutions should be infused within 24 hours.
- Handling
    - Use clean technique when handling enteral solutions.
    - Use aseptic technique when handling parenteral solutions.
- Disposal: dispose of all unused, partially used, or expired materials consistent with local ordinances and conventions; as environmental standards within communities become updated, an annual call to the state health department environmental office is recommended in order to maintain compliant policies and procedures

Goals/Outcomes

- Develop a safe and comfortable environment for patient/caregiver and hospice staff
- Appropriate use of medical equipment, supplies, and medications
- Decrease financial and legal worries concerning patient care issues
- Maintain patient/caregiver preferences and dignity as much as possible, balanced against safe working conditions for professional/volunteer staff

Documentation in the Medical Record

Initial Psychosocial/Practical Assessment

- Environmental assessment, risks, barriers to care
- Determination of support systems
- Definition of financial and legal issues that may affect care

Interdisciplinary Progress Notes

- Instruction in basic safety measures (environmental, medical)
- Summation of discussions regarding options for environmental, financial, legal help and patient/caregiver responses, preferences
- Description of interventions
- Results of interventions

IDT Care Plan

- Description of interventions: who, what, when
- Contingency and follow-up plans and alternatives based upon results of discussions/interventions and patient/caregiver response

Suicide: Risk, Prevention, and Coping If It Happens

SITUATION: Patient expressing thoughts or wishes for self-inflicted/assisted death or suicide occurs

Findings

- Signs and symptoms of severe depression
- Overwhelming sense of hopelessness, meaninglessness, purposelessness, despair
- Expression of death wishes
- Devaluation of life and living
- Suicidal ideation, gestures, plan
- Sense of giving up and giving in (blissful euphoric affect or despair)
- Repeated expressions of being a burden, excessive guilt or shame
- Feelings of being abandoned (by friends, family, God)
- Accrual of large doses of central nervous system-depressant drugs (opioids, hypnotics, sedatives, anxiolytics, etc.)
- Prior history of major depression, impulsive behavior, suicide attempt(s)

Assessment

Biomedical

- Determine whether any physical symptoms are out of control and patient/caregiver beliefs, perceptions about symptom control issues
- Review medications and determine if symptoms may reflect drug-related adverse effect

Psychosocial/Spiritual

- Review prior history of depression, anxiety, absence of coping skills, and suicide attempt(s) and formally assess for signs and symptoms of major depression (refer to the *DSM-IV-TR*)
- Review coexisting social/environmental stresses that may be contributing to sense of despair (separation/divorce, loss of job, income, prestige, etc.)
- Evaluate family/caregiver behaviors that suggest patient is burdensome
- Evaluate beliefs/faith and understand patient's value system (self-view, sense of hope and hopelessness, meaning, purpose, etc.)
- Understand patient's expressed wishes to end life if able to articulate them
- Determine if there is a concrete suicide plan
- • Determine high risk of imminent suicide by presence of:
  - Specific suicide plan.
  - Availability of resources to carry out plan.
  - History of prior suicide attempts.
  - Misuse of medications/alcohol.
  - Hearing voices to kill self.
  - Inadequate social support.
  - Agitation or flat affect coupled with despair.

Processes of Care

Biomedical

- Vigorously treat all out-of-control symptoms
- Initiate antidepressant therapy if indicated and monitor closely

Psychosocial/Spiritual

- Low risk: no plan, no substantial ideation, no significant risk factors
  - Assist in identifying positive aspects of patient's life and areas of "unfinished business."
  - Help to establish attainable short-term goals.
  - Assist in developing and strengthening relationships.
  - Address issues regarding self-image and any distorted thinking.
  - Provide 24-hour contact and consider continuous care if suicidal ideation increases.
  - Offer pastoral care or facilitate involvement with existing spiritual/religious leader.
  - Invite discussions regarding sense of meaning and purpose.
  - Assist in providing activities to assuage boredom.

- Involve family/caregiver in discussions with patient regarding sense of burden.
- Help to arrange respite for family/caregiver as necessary.
- Educate entire IDT as to level of risk and need to monitor for increased risk.
- Moderate to high risk (substantial ideation and plan with significant risk factors, per above)
  - Utilize interventions as described above.
  - Notify physician.
  - Explain limits of professional confidentiality applied to potential suicide.
  - Discuss negative consequences of suicide.
  - Attempt to establish a verbal or written "no suicide contract."
  - Instruct caregiver to observe for changes in mood or behavior and who to notify.
  - Attempt to remove all lethal agents.
  - Provide multiple contacts (crisis line, suicide prevention, hospice, chaplaincy).
  - Daily visits from patient-preferred hospice staff member who has expertise in suicide prevention and management of depression and adjustment reactions.
  - Arrange mental health expert consultation as needed.
- Occurrence of suicide
  - Notify physician for appropriate completion of death certificate.
  - Provide intensive bereavement support and counseling to family/caregiver.
  - Refer family/caregiver to support groups as needed and per family preference.
  - Provide "debriefing" and staff support for IDT members intimately involved in care.

Goals/Outcomes

- Enable patient's sense of purpose and meaning in remaining existence
- Prevent suicide without stripping patient of dignity, autonomy, and rights of self-determination
- Attain closure and functional grieving for family/caregiver and staff if suicide occurs

Documentation in the Medical Record

Initial Biomedical Assessment

- Formal evaluation for symptom control and severe mood disorder

Initial Psychosocial/Spiritual Assessment

- Define level of risk and options discussed.
- Document contributing factors.

Interdisciplinary Team Notes

- Results of discussions, reassessments, and specific interventions
- Documentation of suicide prevention plan and change in level of risk

IDT Care Plan

- Specific interventions and contingency plans (who, what, when)
- Follow-up plan

Section 3

Clinical Processes and Symptom Management

Pain and symptom management is a key focus of hospice care, because it is rare for people who are experiencing severe physical distress to consider other aspects of their existence. Improvements in pharmaceuticals and pharmacotherapy have served to enhance the ability to keep distressing symptoms associated with advanced disease under reasonable control in the vast majority of cases. Therefore, excellence in pharmacotherapy plays a critical role in the provision of high-quality hospice care, so solid grounding in this area is the starting point for the hospice clinician's knowledge base. A fundamental principle is that all medication management must be tailored to the individual needs and situation of the patient. The information provided in this section is meant to guide therapy and should not be used rigidly in lieu of clinical judgment. Pharmacoeconomics always plays a role in current-day health care, so cost considerations will enter into decision-making at some level. These analyses should be used in order to make balanced decisions after sound assessment principles have been followed, leading to an indication for a therapeutic intervention.

Knowledgeable clinicians recognize that many symptoms (e.g., pain, anxiety, restlessness) have an often-lengthy differential diagnosis. For example, restlessness may reflect metabolic encephalopathy, air hunger (dyspnea), hypoxia, pain that is poorly localized or difficult to express, social stress, an unresolved emotional or spiritual issue, and so forth. Furthermore, each of these etiologies has its own lengthy differential diagnosis that may require further evaluation and specific treatment.

It is always incumbent on the clinician to make the best determination of the CAUSE of the distressing symptom in order to promote the best PALLIATION of the symptom. The more closely these are matched, the more likely it is that the patient's (and caregiver's) needs will be met. With this in mind, pharmacotherapy may not always be the best approach to symptom management. When it is, this guide should serve as a means of making this process more uniform and timely, actualizing the goals of maximizing therapeutic effect and minimizing adverse effects. Careful titration of drugs, especially when using polypharmacy (more than one drug at a time), is required to avoid toxic effects, especially when drug–drug interactions and synergistic effects are likely to occur. These should be understood, anticipated, prevented, and monitored. The effects of aging amplify many drug effects, and these principles and precautions should be accentuated in older individuals.

Because many symptom and treatment domains are overlapping (e.g., dysphagia and painful mucositis) cross-referencing will serve to make this resource as useful and compact as possible. When issues are not crystal clear, we can and should rely on the strength, diversity, and breadth of experience within the interdisciplinary team to find direction. True emergencies (e.g., pain out of control, extreme agitation, severe dyspnea) should trigger immediate intervention and, when necessary, consultation. For medically oriented problems, this guide should serve as a reference for immediate action, to relieve suffering as quickly as possible.

Clinicians should always choose the drug formulation that is believed to best serve the patient's needs, after all pertinent variables have been considered. Although clinical experience is invaluable, reliance on anecdotal experience alone is a dangerous trap. Generally speaking, extemporaneous formulations (compounding) should be avoided in favor of commercial formulations, because the latter are subject to considerable regulatory scrutiny and quality control, so factors such as dissolution and absorption are far more likely to be predictable. Last, expense is always a consideration in health care, and hospice in particular, due to its payment structure under the Medicare Hospice Benefit. Cost-effective therapies should drive clinical decision-making, not cost containment. Good business practices combined with skilled case management should allow all patients to obtain the most beneficial treatments available in order to optimize therapeutic outcomes.

Air Hunger (Dyspnea)

SITUATION: Shortness of breath, chest tightness, and air hunger are often associated with findings of anxiety, panic, desperation, or impending doom.

This symptom is often more distressing than pain. Although it is very important to formulate a differential diagnosis as quickly as possible in order to match treatment with the identified cause whenever possible, **never delay palliative treatment for any reason.** Air hunger is probably the most terrifying symptom that can be experienced, and panic can overcome even the most stable and well-prepared patient, family, and other caregivers. THE EMERGENT TREATMENT OF CHOICE IS MORPHINE (OR ANOTHER RAPID-ONSET OPIOID IF THERE IS MORPHINE ALLERGY/SENSITIVITY), UNLESS A CAUSE IS IMMEDIATELY IDENTIFIED THAT CAN BE TREATED JUST AS QUICKLY. **ALTHOUGH BRONCHOSPASM, CONGESTIVE HEART FAILURE, AND OTHER CAUSES MAY ALSO REQUIRE EMERGENT TREATMENT, OPIOIDS SHOULD BE GIVEN CONCURRENTLY OR SHORTLY AFTER MEDICATIONS FOR THESE OTHER SPECIFIC CONDITIONS ARE GIVEN.** Fear of hypercapnia is often cited as a reason to delay use of opioids, but the literature consistently supports the safety of opioid use in dyspnea, when used at appropriate doses. The most rapid, readily accessible, and immediately available route of administration for morphine should be used.

For emergent/urgent treatment, choices include the following:

- Oral morphine concentrate (20 mg/ml): 1/4 to 1/2 ml (5 to 10 mg) sublingual (SL)/oral (PO); repeat in 15–30 minutes as needed. May need higher doses in people with opioid tolerance, just as in pain management, and can use other opioids (for equianalgesic doses see "Pain" later in this section). Dose of opioids for prn use when tolerance is present is 10% to 15% of usual total 24-hour opioid dosage.

- Nebulized morphine (parenteral grade, preservative free) 2.5 mg in 2 to 4 ml 0.9% (normal) saline or fentanyl 25 to 50 μg (1/2 to 1 ml) in the same volume of saline is an alternative if more readily available or if there is morphine sensitivity.
- Parenteral opioid delivery via the subcutaneous (SQ) route is feasible in most settings.

For patients who have established intravenous (IV) access, it may be preferable and faster to titrate IV morphine, starting with 1 mg every few minutes in opioid-naïve patients, or an equivalent opioid (e.g., 10 μg fentanyl; 0.15 mg hydromorphone).

- The dose of opioid, regardless of route of administration, should be adjusted based on the previous experience and opioid tolerance of the patient.
- Benzodiazepines can also be used as adjuvants to opioids. Liquid lorazepam (2 mg/ml) can be given at a dose of 0.25 to 0.5 ml (0.5 to 1 mg) and repeated in 30 minutes as needed. Some studies have shown benzodiazepines to be equivalent or even superior to opioids in relieving dyspnea.

Causes

Practical

- Excessive or poorly regulated activity (pacing issues)
- Improper physical positioning (e.g., orthopnea)

Psychosocial/Spiritual

- Anxiety associated with dyspnea itself—i.e., a vicious cycle—or anxiety from other sources of worry, angst, etc., serving as a trigger for dyspnea
- Fear (usually compounded by experiences from previous episodes)
- Undertreated pain can cause anxiety, tachypnea, and dyspnea

Biomedical

- Pulmonary disease (e.g., chronic obstructive pulmonary disease [COPD], restrictive lung disease, pneumonia)
- Pleural effusion
- Pericardial effusion
- Neuromuscular disease affecting coordinated mechanics of breathing and respiratory muscle function
- Uncompensated heart failure
- Weakness, fatigue, aesthenia due to primary disease or secondary causes (e.g., metabolic derangement, myasthenia)
- Anemia with inadequate oxygen-carrying capacity
- Acute pulmonary embolism (PE)
- Acute myocardial infarction (MI)

Findings

- Anxiety, restlessness, fearfulness, agitation, "panic facies"
- Complaint of shortness of breath or similar expression of breathing difficulties
- Inability to speak in complete sentences due to running out of breath
- Decreased functional ability due to shortness of breath
- Increased use of accessory muscles of respiration and posturing to catch breath (head forward, pursed-lip breathing, sitting bolt upright)
- Tachypnea
- Cyanosis, hypoxemia

Assessment

Practical

- Air circulation
- Dust, pollen, pet hair, strong perfumes/cleansers, etc.
- Patient positioning, availability of pillows, bolsters, etc.
- Assess bowel habits/constipation/stool impaction, especially if opioids are being used
- Proximity of medications, caregiver
- Knowledge and understanding of crisis prevention plan

Biomedical

- Review diagnosis and likely medical etiologies for symptoms
- Vital signs (respiratory rate, pattern, depth; pulse rate and quality; blood pressure [BP]; temperature)
- Cardiac examination: rate, rhythm, peripheral perfusion, venous distention
- Pulmonary examination: quality of breath sounds (wheezes, rales, rhonchi/rattles, acute changes)
- Extremity examination: edema, skin turgor, pallor
- Abdominal examination: acute distention, ascites, tenderness
- Check oxygen saturation (portable pulse oximeter) for acute changes
- Patient self-rating of intensity/severity of episode(s) using a standardized numerical (0 to 10) scale (verbal or visual, depending on patient preference and capability) with 0 being "no shortness of breath" and 10 being "worst shortness of breath imaginable"; repeat measurements should be taken and noted after intervention(s); link patient/caregiver self-care and crisis prevention/intervention plan to severity ratings after some experience with this type of tool
- Occasionally, laboratory evaluation of hemoglobin/hematocrit to determine potential causes of limited oxygen-carrying capacity may be necessary if first-line palliative measures are not proving to be effective

Psychosocial/Spiritual

- Acquire history of previous experiences, interventions, worries, plan for preventing crises, and potential emotional triggering factors

Processes of Care

Practical

- Avoid gas-forming foods to prevent gastric/bowel distention
- Discuss and facilitate remedial environmental adjustments to decrease symptom triggers and improve respiratory mechanics (e.g., rest periods, pacing, raise head of bed, use of bolsters, etc.)
- Instruct patient/caregiver in optimum patient positioning, day and night
- Provide durable medical equipment (DME) as needed for positioning
- Provide air movement using a fan and/or humidifier if at all possible and determine symptomatic utility
- Teach percussion and vibration to caregiver(s) as indicated
- Devise crisis prevention and care plan
- Review regularly: what to do, when and who to call
- Check patient/caregiver understanding
- Optimize accessibility and availability of prophylactic/therapeutic/communication resources

Biomedical

- Notify physician of any unexpected or significant changes in physical examination that may require change in care plan or physician evaluation
- Institute oxygen therapy ONLY if demonstrated that patient is hypoxemic AND there is a therapeutic response to the use of supplemental oxygen. Otherwise, use personal fans or other means of increasing air circulation
- Optimize medical management (diuretics, vasodilators, bronchodilators)
- Consider trial of passive positive pressure (external) breathing device, if available
- Palliative pharmacotherapy
  - Primarily anxiety-triggered dyspnea:
    — Anxiolytic therapy: lorazepam PO/SL/SQ 0.5 to 2 mg q2–4hr or prn is given.
    — *NOTE: Titrate dose slowly to effect, especially when using in combination with opioids, to determine patient's sensitivity.*
  - Primarily non–anxiety-triggered dyspnea:
    — Opioid therapy: rapidity of onset and therapeutic effect is a function of establishing blood levels as quickly as possible.
    — For patients with IV access, titrate IV doses to effect q15 min (e.g., morphine sulfate 1 mg or equivalent) to determine patient's sensitivity and threshold for response.
    — For patients without IV access, similar SQ doses can be given, or administer oral morphine concentrate (20 mg/ml) titrated to effect, starting with 0.25 to 0.5 ml SL/PO. Alternatively, nebulized morphine 2.5 mg in 2 to 4 ml 0.9% (normal) saline or fentanyl 25 to 50 µg in the same volume of saline is recommended. The medical literature is inconclusive about this form of therapy, but anecdotal experience

has been favorable in some patients, especially as an alternative to establishing IV access or much slower absorption routes (SQ/SL). This symptom should be anticipated in susceptible patients so that the apparatus for nebulizer treatments is readily available.

— An alternative to nebulized or parenteral drug delivery in order to establish rapid patient-controlled levels of opioid is fentanyl via the buccal or SL route. Various formulations are available, as either a lozenge on a stick, dissolvable tablets (buccal and sublingual), buccal patches, or a nasal spray. It is recommended to start at the lowest available dose (100 or 200 μg) ONLY IN OPIOID-TOLERANT PATIENTS; this provides opioid-tolerant patients a noninvasive, self-administered means of relieving dyspnea for those without IV access, SQ dosing, or immediate access to nebulizer set-up. There is limited clinical experience with this technique.

— Recurrent episodic therapy with opioid analgesics by the most convenient route with an anxiolytic (lorazepam PO/SL/SQ 0.5 to 2 mg q2–4hr or prn) is usually necessary until death unless there is a well-defined remediable cause (see below).

Treatable Causes

1. Bronchospasm: A history of asthma or COPD is usually present. Listen for expiratory wheezes. Use a nebulized β_2-agonist (e.g., albuterol). Inhaled corticosteroids (e.g., beclomethasone) are proving to be beneficial in relieving acute bronchospasm. Systemic corticosteroids (e.g., prednisone) may be required in refractory cases.

2. Pulmonary edema: Volume overload and left ventricular failure, leading to right ventricular failure, are the most common causes. Restriction of fluids and limiting sodium intake (or artificial feedings) and use of morphine therapy may relieve acute symptoms. In refractory cases, consider initiating or advancing diuretic therapy (furosemide 40 to 240 mg), inotropic therapy (digoxin), and angiotensin-converting enzyme (ACE) inhibitor therapy, according to clinical signs and symptoms, assessed by auscultation of heart and lungs, jugular venous distention, peripheral edema, and balance of fluid intake and (urinary) output.

   In severe cases, where urgent palliation is indicated, parenteral diuretic and opioid drug administration is warranted, by the most convenient route (IV, IM).

3. Bronchial obstruction by tumor: Consider radiation therapy if prognosis allows; corticosteroid therapy for end-stage palliation (e.g., dexamethasone up to 12 mg/day in divided doses); and for symptomatic relief, nebulized fentanyl and lidocaine have also been used with varying degrees of efficacy.

4. Pleural effusion: Consider thoracentesis only if symptoms are not readily managed by noninvasive means (opioid and benzodiazepine pharmacotherapy, positioning, diuretics) and there is likelihood of significant improvement in performance status or return to a level of functioning

meaningful to the patient. In the final days of life, thoracentesis (especially if not able to be performed in the home) adds a greater burden than benefit. If nonloculated peripheral pleural effusions recur within days, and the relief of symptoms was viewed as meaningful to the patient, consideration for pleurodesis is appropriate in patients with a life expectancy of more than a few weeks.

5. Superior vena cava syndrome (obstruction of the superior vena cava): dexamethasone 24 mg IV followed by aggressive symptom control with corticosteroid, opioid, and benzodiazepine pharmacotherapy while considering the merits of radiation therapy (for patients with an otherwise predicted life expectancy of more than a few weeks).

6. Ascites: Diuretic therapy (e.g., furosemide 40 mg PO and spironolactone 100 mg PO per day, titrated upward as needed to maximum daily doses of furosemide 240 mg, spironolactone 400 mg) is the first line of therapy. However, diuretics are rarely helpful in cases of malignant ascites. In terminal disease states, paracentesis is rarely indicated. In cases of slowly developing ascites leading to dyspnea, where the burdens of symptom-relieving pharmacotherapy (opioids plus benzodiazepines) seem to outweigh the benefits, paracentesis should be considered if there is a life expectancy of several days to weeks.

7. Secretory conditions: Consider scopolamine SQ (0.2 to 0.4 mg) or transdermal; or glycopyrrolate 0.2 mg SQ and saline nebulizer treatments.

Psychosocial

- Teach relaxation techniques, cognitive-behavioral techniques, and breathing exercises
- Address worries and fears in a direct, supportive way; help solve problems when concrete issues arise
- Reduce anxiety by assuring patient and caregiver that measures to improve symptoms will be taken immediately

Goals/Outcomes

- Reduced frequency and intensity of dyspneic episodes, with concurrent decrease in distress
- Improved sleep, appetite (if applicable), social interaction, mood, interest in what life has to offer
- Improved functional status (if applicable) (e.g., self-care, time out of bed, toileting out of bed, etc.)
- Decreased work of breathing
- Elimination of crises and unwanted interventions and transfers (e.g., ambulance calls, emergency department visits, hospitalizations, intubation, etc.)

Documentation in the Medical Record

Initial Medical Assessment

- Pertinent systemic review, examination findings, diagnostic impressions
- Dyspnea rating (patient self-report)

Initial Practical/Psychosocial/Spiritual Assessment

- Nonmedical initiating and contributing factors

Interdisciplinary Progress Notes

- Results of interventions
- Changes in biomedical, psychosocial, spiritual issues and circumstances influencing symptoms and management
- Repeat dyspnea ratings (patient self-report)

IDT Care Plan

- Nonpharmacological and pharmacological interventions with appropriate medical orders
- Follow-up and contingency plans
- Crisis prevention/intervention plan

Recommended Reading

Abernethy AP, McDonald CF, Frith PA, et al. Effect of palliative oxygen versus room air in relief of breathlessness in patients with refractory dyspnoea: a double-blind, randomised controlled trial. Lancet. 2010;376(9743):784–793

Clemens KE, Quednau I, Klaschik E. Use of oxygen and opioids in the palliation of dyspnoea in hypoxic and non-hypoxic palliative care patients: a prospective study. Support Care Cancer. 2009;17(4):367–377

Cranston JM, Crockett A, Currow D. Oxygen therapy for dyspnoea in adults. Cochrane Database Syst Rev. 2008 Jul 16;(3):CD004769

Currow DC, Agar M, Smith J, Abernethy AP. Does palliative home oxygen improve dyspnoea? A consecutive cohort study. Palliat Med. 2009;23(4):309–316

Currow DC, Smith J, Davidson PM et al. Do the trajectories of dyspnea differ in prevalence and intensity by diagnosis a the end of life? A consecutive cohort study. J Pain Symptom Manage. 2010;39(4):680–690

Mahler DA, Selecky PA, Harrod CG, Benditt JO, et al. American College of Chest Physicians consensus statement on the management of dyspnea in patients with advanced lung or heart disease. Chest 2010;137(3):674–691

Naviganti AH, Castro MA, Cerchietti LC. Morphine versus midazolam as upfront therapy to control dyspnea perception in cancer patients while its underlying cause is sought or treated. J Pain Symptom Manage. 2010;39(5):820–330

Agitation and Anxiety

SITUATION: Anxiety or agitation that is distressing to the patient/ caregiver or negatively affects care of the patient or the caregiving environment

Severe anxiety (or panic) and uncontrolled agitation represent some of the few, but true, emergency conditions (along with convulsions, hemorrhage, severe dyspnea and pain) in the hospice setting. Anticipation and early recognition of these circumstances with a prevention and treatment plan are critical to optimum care of the dying.

Causes

Biomedical

- Respiratory distress (e.g., dyspnea from any cause; symptomatic hypoxemia and/or hypercarbia)
- Uncontrolled pain
- Primary anxiety/panic disorder
- Disease-induced psychosis (e.g., brain metastasis, metabolic disturbance)
- Drug-related psychosis (e.g., opioids, corticosteroids, medications with anti-cholinergic side effects)
- Sleep deprivation
- Agitated depression
- Full bladder, fecal impaction, nausea in a patient who cannot express distress other than through behavioral response
- Substance abuse/misuse/withdrawal (e.g., alcohol, opioid, benzodiazepine abstinence syndrome)

Psychosocial/Spiritual

- Response to imminent loss (anticipatory grief)
- Fear of the unknown and other fears associated with severe illness and imminent death
- Nightmares/night terrors

Findings

- Verbal or other expressions of anxiety, panic, terror, fear, worry
- Disordered sleep
- Misuse of prescribed medications and noncompliance with other treatment protocols
- Abusive language or behaviors toward caregivers
- Push of speech, tangential thoughts, perseveration
- Volatile behavior; combative behavior
- Altered appetite
- Somatization
- "Panic" behaviors (e.g., frequent impulsive telephone calls, dialing 911)
- Increased complaints of pain that are not responsive to analgesic medication management
- Autonomic nervous system reactions (tachycardia, diaphoresis, tachypnea)
- Sense of impending doom or death without accompanying biomedical signs

NOTE: In advanced disease states, especially cancer, differentiating physical symptoms due to anxiety from those attributable to somatic, visceral, or neurogenic manifestations of the disease may be extremely difficult. Empirical therapy may be required.

Evaluation

Biomedical

- Evaluate for concomitant evidence suggesting an organic brain syndrome due to advancing disease with either local or systemic manifestations (e.g., hallucinations, nausea/vomiting, papilledema, hypo/hyperglycemia, uremia)

NOTE: Laboratory testing should be done only if findings will specifically alter or influence the plan of care to alleviate distressing symptoms.

- Review medications for adverse drug reactions (e.g., psychotropic drugs, analgesics, corticosteroids, medications with anticholinergic side effects)
- Ensure that all medications whose abrupt discontinuation can lead to an acute abstinence syndrome are either maintained or slowly tapered

NOTE: Consult with physician or pharmacist for dosage conversion and formulations if an alternative route of administration is necessary.

- Conduct systems review and examination of bladder and bowel function (e.g., urinary retention, constipation, impaction)
- Examine less-than-fully coherent or noncommunicative patients for signs of unrecognized pain source (e.g., bone pain, abdominal pain, decubitus pain, etc.)
- Respiratory examination for potential cause of hypoxemia/dyspnea (respiratory rate and pattern, use of accessory muscles, pallor/cyanosis, rales, pleural effusion)
- Cardiac examination for evidence of heart failure, ischemia or arrhythmia (rate, rhythm, jugular venous distention, peripheral edema, rales, diaphoresis)

Psychosocial/Spiritual

- Patient self-rating on anxiety scale (if capable)
- Caregiver rating of patient on agitation scale
- Assess patient/caregiver perceptions of cause/source of anxiety/agitation
- Review past experiences with significant losses and deaths
- Review current and past history of anxiety/panic disorder and psychiatric care; refer to *Diagnostic Statistical Manual, Fourth Edition (DSM-IV-TR)* for diagnostic criteria
- Identify coping skills/social support and barriers to care
- Observe interactions among caregiver(s)/patient
- Assess impact of anxiety/agitation on overall care
- Identify areas of unresolved conflict

Processes of Care

Biomedical

- If hypoxemia-induced agitation responds to a trial of oxygen therapy, maintain oxygen administration protocol with usual recommendations and precautions
- Attempt to reduce dyspnea by increasing air circulation with a portable fan

- Listening-talking therapy should precede or supplement pharmacotherapy unless symptoms are immediately uncontrollable or at crisis levels
- Nightmares or terrifying hallucinations and severe anxiety or agitation should be controlled emergently for the patient's and family's sake

Pharmacotherapy for acute and recurrent anxiety

1. Lorazepam 0.5 mg PO/SL/SQ/IV q2–4hr; titrate dose and interval as needed; oral formulations of lorazepam (PO/SL) are considerably less costly than parenteral formulations; sublingual lorazepam has been shown to be absorbed (attain plasma levels) similarly to parenteral administration

2. In a crisis, without IV access, subcutaneous injection of lorazepam (1 to 2 mg) is the most expedient means to attain a calm setting in which to seek out more specific treatment approaches (complete the assessment) or institute longer-term maintenance therapy

3. Patients who are not responsive to low- or moderate-dose benzodiazepine therapy require further evaluation

4. Patients who are responsive to low- or moderate-dose benzodiazepine therapy and who continue to have anxiety and have a prognosis of weeks to months may benefit from a daily antidepressant—e.g., SSRI (selective serotonin reuptake inhibitor such as paroxetine), SNRI (serotonin-norepinephrine reuptake inhibitor such as venlafaxine), or buspirone

Pharmacotherapy for acute and recurrent agitation

1. Mild or moderate restlessness or delirium: haloperidol 0.5 to 5 mg PO/SQ/IV q4–6hr (titrate upward as needed) or chlorpromazine 10 mg IV or 25 mg PO/PR q6–8hr (titrate upward as needed; SQ chlorpromazine should not be given because of skin irritation, risk of necrosis)

2. More severe delirium and terminal restlessness (involuntary movements) often require more rapid dose titration and combination therapy; paradoxical reactions to sedative drugs can occur; these effects should be recognized quickly so that alternative therapies can be instituted.

   a. Start with above-noted therapies (haloperidol or chlorpromazine plus lorazepam). If this is ineffective, consider adding pentobarbital suppository 60 to 120 mg PR q4hr as needed. Diphenhydramine 25 to 50 mg PO/IV q6hr should be used if extrapyramidal effects are noted when using haloperidol or chlorpromazine (avoid these drugs in patients with Parkinson's disease).

   b. An expensive but effective alternative for control of terminal agitation symptoms that are poorly responsive to first-line therapies above is SQ/IV midazolam. It can be first given as a bolus dose of 5 mg followed by a continuous infusion of 1 mg/hr. Titrate up or down according to level of consciousness and emergence of symptoms. If a continuous infusion is not (immediately) possible, consider using a SQ port and administrating midazolam SQ q2–4hr scheduled or prn.

   c. Another costly but effective treatment for total sedation in an inpatient setting is propofol infusion. This requires a functional IV line and the supervision of a clinician experienced in the management of total sedation using this technique. Usual doses for initiating therapy are 10-mg (1-ml) incremental boluses in rapid succession (q1–5min, depending on patient's circulation time) until effective sedation versus respiratory function is achieved. Continuous infusion at a rate of 10 to 50 µg/kg/hr is usually the effective range, but this must be titrated to individual circumstances and response. Propofol can be painful when infused through a peripheral vein. The addition of preservative-free lidocaine in a ratio of 40 mg lidocaine: 200 mg propofol (1 ml 4% lidocaine added to each 20 ml propofol) is effective in eliminating pain during bolus or infusion.

Psychosocial/Spiritual

- Teach relaxation, imaging, and distraction techniques when applicable
- Openly discuss feelings, perceptions, role changes, losses, and issues of control and frustration
- Interact with patient/caregiver in a calm, reassuring manner
- Use life review and storytelling techniques to engage patient and discern sources of conflict
- Acknowledge and reduce fears and worries by providing information and clarifying distortions in thinking in a gentle and sensitive manner:
  - What can the patient/caregiver expect over the next days to weeks?
  - What is usual course of the disease and prognosis?
- Be open and invite all questions; look for the meaning behind "cloaked" questions
- Reinforce coping skills and anxiety-reducing behaviors/techniques
- Facilitate problem-solving and decision-making
- Provide instruction on how to create a calm environment for patient and caregiver (be aware that paradoxical effects may occur—some people prefer chaos):
  - Reduce noise, bright light, clutter.
  - Increase structure, schedules, orderliness.
  - Limit physical restraints.
- Design crisis intervention plan for emergency management of out-of-control symptoms
- Have pharmacotherapy orders available (see above under "Biomedical")
- Have hospice on-call telephone number immediately available
- Hospice staff to consult with physician if symptoms do not respond to interventions within reasonable time period (1 to 4 hours, depending on severity of symptoms)

Goals/Outcomes

- Episodes of anxiety/agitation will be reduced in frequency and intensity in order to reduce both distress to the patient and caregiver burden

- To provide an opportunity for reconciling internal and interpersonal conflicts
- To eliminate the likelihood of self-harm or injury to caregivers
- To prevent avoidable transfers and discontinuity in care setting whenever possible

Documentation in the Medical Record

Initial Psychosocial/Spiritual Assessment

- Anxiety score recorded using standard analog scale (patient report)
- Agitation score recorded using standard analog scale (caregiver report)
- Manifestations of anxiety/agitation
- Ability of caregiver to cope with patient's condition
- Social/environmental factors that contribute to anxiety/agitation

Initial Medical Assessment

- Medical findings and contributors to anxiety/agitation
- Physical manifestations of anxiety/agitation
- Effects of anxiety/agitation on medical condition
- Current medication and other substance use for pain, insomnia, restlessness, anxiety/agitation

Interdisciplinary Progress Notes

- Anxiety score recorded using 0-to-10 scale (patient report)
- Agitation score recorded using 0-to-10 scale (caregiver report)
- Patient/caregiver response to proposed interventions (e.g., agreement, denial, defensiveness, disregard, anger, etc.)
- Patient/caregiver compliance/acceptance of care plan
- Results of interventions and reassessments

IDT Care Plan

- Proposed interventions: who, when, what
- Contingency plans and reassessment schedule
- Crisis prevention/intervention plan

Recommended Reading

Breitbart W. A double-blind trial of haloperidol, chlorpromazine and lorazepam in the treatment of delirium in hospitalized AIDS patients. Am J Psychiatry. 1996;153(2):231–237

Casarett DJ, Inouye SK. Diagnosis and management of delirium near the end of life. Ann Intern Med. 2001;135:32–40

Lawlor PG, Fainsinger RL, Bruera ED. Delirium at the end of life. JAMA. 2000; 284(19):2427–2429

Palliative Care Medications Commonly Used Subcutaneously. www.palliative.org/ PC/ClinicalInfo/scchartFeb05.pdf

White C, et al. First do no harm … Terminal restlessness or drug-induced delirium. J Palliat Med. 2007;10(2):345–351

Anorexia and Cachexia

SITUATION: Progressive decline in appetite, nutritional status, and body mass as a result of catabolic changes associated with chronic disease

Approximately 80% of people with advanced disease suffer from these debilitating and often demoralizing consequences of cancer and other chronic disease states. Despite the high prevalence of hospice patients who are affected by anorexia and cachexia, uniform definitions of these often-coexisting conditions have not been agreed upon. Clinically useful definitions for the hospice clinician include:

- Anorexia is the uncontrolled lack or loss of appetite for food
- Cachexia is involuntary weight loss
  - The evolving definition of cachexia further refines this to loss of muscle with or without loss of fat mass.
  - It is becoming more evident that cancer anorexia-cachexia syndrome (CACS) appears to be a distinct disorder with unique clinical characteristics. Because of the rapid rate of change in the characterization of this syndrome, emerging diagnostic and treatment options, and the dramatic, negative impact on quality of life for patients, it is important that the hospice clinician remains abreast of these developments in the years to come.

Causes

Biomedical

- Cancer
  - Especially common in tumors of the head and neck, gastrointestinal tract, pancreas, central nervous system, and lungs
- Cardiac disease
- Chronic kidney disease
- Chronic obstructive pulmonary disease
- HIV/AIDS
- Rheumatoid arthritis

Findings

- Decreased or no appetite with lack of interest in eating
- Feeling of fullness after minimal ingestion of food (early satiety) that may result from organomegaly ("squashed stomach")
- Continuous underlying presence of nausea
- Changes in taste perception, often unpleasant
- Dehydration, uremia, hypercalcemia, and other metabolic alterations
- Oral candidiasis, mucositis
- Gastritis

Evaluation

Practical

- Environmental assessment to determine source(s) of unpleasant odors
- Determine food preferences, reactions to various foods (what is particularly pleasant/unpleasant) and recent food intake, patterns of hunger/eating

if any, and practical limitations such as ability to chew, swallow, use of dentures, etc.

- Determine patient/caregiver understanding and capability to prepare modified foods (e.g., blended, pureed), if there are barriers to obtaining foods (e.g., transportation, finances), and any practical limitations of food storage or preparation (e.g., refrigeration, cooking, infestation)

Biomedical

- Identify underlying causes or contributing factors that may be subject to palliation, correction, or treatment if the patient's sense of well-being is negatively affected by signs/symptoms:
  - Pain
  - Nausea
  - Uremia, hypercalcemia
  - Constipation, obstipation, impaction
  - Bowel obstruction
  - Hepatomegaly
  - Depression
  - Oral candidiasis
  - Mucositis, esophagitis, gastritis
  - Xerostomia (dry mouth)
- Assess patient's ability to swallow
- Though not in widespread use, CT scans are an important new tool in the diagnosis of the anorexia-cachexia syndrome
  - CT data may reveal sarcopenia (severe muscle wasting). This is most commonly evaluated by measuring skeletal muscle cross-sectional area at L3. Sarcopenia is a particularly important finding, as studies have shown links between sarcopenia and functional status, chemotherapy toxicity, time to tumor progression, and mortality.

Psychosocial/Spiritual

- Assess symbolic value of nutrition/hydration to patient/caregiver (nurturing, guilt) and identify areas of patient/caregiver conflicting opinions, beliefs, or values related to feeding/hydration
- Determine to what degree anorexia/cachexia signs and symptoms are disturbing to patient/caregiver and what preferences/goals/concerns exist about these

Processes of Care

Practical

- Facilitate means to reduce environmental factors that negatively influence patient's interest/enjoyment in meals and suggest enhancements such as:
  - Provide a preprandial alcoholic beverage of choice, if acceptable and tolerated.
  - Make an effort to take meals in esthetically pleasing environment with companionship rather than in bed or sleeping area.

- Have patient suck on hard candy (trial and error of sweet versus sour/citrus) to mask bad tastes.
- Involve patient in menu planning.
- Try very small portions with more frequent feedings, if patient is interested.
- Suggest cold (semi-frozen) nutritional drinks to overcome difficulties with chewing, swallowing, and odor/taste aberrations if patient is interested.

Biomedical

- Inform patient/caregiver of relative risks/burdens versus benefits of various routes of alimentation and hydration as applicable
- Palliative pharmacotherapy (in order of demonstrated efficacy)

1. Corticosteroids
   a. Dexamethasone 1 to 2 mg PO tid
   b. Methylprednisolone 1 to 2 mg PO bid
   c. Prednisone 5 mg PO tid
2. Hormonal therapy
   a. Megestrol acetate 80 to 160 mg PO qid
3. Other approaches
   a. Dronabinol 2.5 mg PO bid to tid
   b. Cyproheptadine 8 mg PO tid
   c. Thalidomide has been found to reduce anorexia/cachexia associated with HIV disease, although it is very costly compared with other available medications
   d. Immunomodulators are a new class of medications being tested in the treatment of anorexia-cachexia; results of early clinical trials have shown significant improvements in anorexia, dyspepsia, strength, and depression; although not yet available for routine clinical use, these agents may prove invaluable in improving the quality of life of palliative care patients in the foreseeable future

Psychosocial/Spiritual

- Reassure patient/caregiver/family that anorexia/cachexia are usual occurrences associated with progressive chronic diseases
- Help open up discussion regarding any conflicts that may exist concerning nutrition and hydration
- Educate and dispel myths about utility of alimentation (enteral or parenteral) under conditions of "wasting" diseases
- Discuss ethical/moral concerns regarding alimentation and hydration in the face of life-limiting illness
- The Macmillan approach to weight and eating is a new psychosocial intervention for weight- and eating-related distress in people with advanced disease states (primarily cancer) and is designed to complement the existing pharmacological and nutritional interventions for cachexia (see http://learnzone.macmillan.org.uk/)

Goals/Outcomes

- Amount, frequency, and type of alimentation/hydration will be commensurate with attainable preferences/goals of patient and appropriate to disease state
- Decrease symptoms attributing to or associated with anorexia/cachexia that are disturbing to patient

Documentation in the Medical Record

Initial Practical/Psychosocial/Spiritual Assessment

- Findings related to environmental factors contributing to troublesome symptoms
- Elaboration of issues pertaining to preferences, goals, and values related to alimentation/hydration; copy and place specific advance directives in chart

Initial Medical Assessment

- Review of systems and history pertaining to and associated with anorexia/cachexia
- Physical findings, stage of disease, nutritional status
- If available, CT images may yield helpful information

Interdisciplinary Progress Notes

- Description of interventions
- Results of interventions
- Ongoing evaluation of mental and physical status

IDT Care Plan

- Goals/outcomes
- Timing of interventions, visits, and contingency plans
- Medical orders for pharmacotherapy

Recommended Reading

Chasen M, Hirschman SZ, Bhargava R. Phase II study of the novel peptide-nucleic acid OHR118 in the management of cancer-related anorexia/cachexia. J Am Med Dir Assoc. 2011;12(1):62–67

Gabison R, Gibbs M, Uziely B, Ganz FD. The Cachexia Assessment Scale: development and psychometric properties. Oncol Nurs Forum. 2010;37(5):635–640

Granda-Cameron C, DeMille D, Lynch MP, Huntzinger C, Alcorn T, Levicoff J, Roop C, Mintzer D. An interdisciplinary approach to manage cancer cachexia. Clin J Oncol Nurs. 2010;14(1):72–80

Holmes S. A difficult clinical problem: diagnosis, impact and clinical management of cachexia in palliative care. Int J Palliat Nurs. 2009;15(7):322–326

Hopkinson JB, Fenlon DR, Okamoto I, Wright DN, Scott I, Addington-Hall JM, Foster C. The deliverability, acceptability, and perceived effect of the Macmillan approach to weight loss and eating difficulties: a phase II, cluster-randomized, exploratory trial of a psychosocial intervention for weight- and eating-related distress in people with advanced cancer. J Pain Symptom Manage. 2010;40(5):684–695

Kwang AY, Kandiah M. Objective and subjective nutritional assessment of patients with cancer in palliative care. Am J Hosp Palliat Care. 2010;27(2):117–126

Prado CM, Birdsell LA, Baracos VE. The emerging role of computerized tomography in assessing cancer cachexia. Curr Opin Support Palliat Care. 2009;3(4):269–275

Belching and Burping (Eructation)

SITUATION: Distress or discomfort associated with frequent belching or persistent gastric distention

Causes

Biomedical

- Aerophagia (air swallowing; may be secondary to anxiety)
- Supra-gastric belching (swallowing air into esophagus and immediately belching, often repetitive)
- Dysfunctional swallowing (cranial nerve or motor impairment)
- Gastric reflux/indigestion
- Gastroparesis, ileus, or small bowel obstruction
- Excessive oral secretions or difficulty managing secretions

Psychosocial

- Anxiety

Findings

Biomedical

- Feeling of epigastric or substernal fullness/pressure; excessive pressure may refer pain to chest or cause esophageal reflux with symptoms of "heartburn"
- Nausea/vomiting
- Abdominal distention (tympany; diminished or excessive bowel sounds [borborygmos])
- Oral lesions and/or excessive secretions
- Impaired swallowing

Psychosocial

- Anxiety state
- Embarrassment
- Social isolation

Evaluation

Biomedical

- Review nutritional status and food intake as cause of excessive gas production (carbonated beverages, dairy products)
- Assess and rule out bowel dysmotility
- Examine oropharynx, cranial nerves, and swallowing action

Psychosocial

- Patient self-rating on anxiety scale (if capable)
- Caregiver rating of patient on agitation scale
- Determine the degree of distress symptoms are causing patient and family; this will help determine how aggressively symptom management should be approached

- Assess patient/caregiver perceptions of cause/source of anxiety/agitation if these emotional factors are believed to be contributory
- Identify coping skills/social support and barriers to care
- Observe interactions among caregiver(s)/patient
- Assess impact of symptoms on overall ability to meet other care goals

Processes of Care

Biomedical

- Evidence of bowel obstruction or ileus should be immediately brought to the attention of the physician before instituting any other therapy
- Mild to moderate symptoms may be reduced by using carbonated beverages to induce air elimination (best to try in presence of staff so that results can be evaluated; discontinue immediately if symptoms worsen)
- Adjust positioning in bed to elevate head to at least 30 degrees
- Dietary instruction to avoid foods that cause indigestion or are difficult to chew and swallow; encourage smaller, more frequent meals
- Instruct patient to thoroughly chew simethicone tablets, if able
- Pharmacotherapy
  1. Simethicone 80-mg chewable tablets before every meal and at HS as needed.
  2. Consider trial of H2 blocker or proton pump inhibitor (PPI).
  3. For anxiety-related symptoms, refer to "Agitation and Anxiety" earlier in this section.
  4. For related oropharyngeal problems, refer to "Dysphagia and Oropharyngeal Problems" later in this section.

Psychosocial

- Teach relaxation, imaging, and distraction techniques when applicable
- Reinforce coping skills and anxiety-reducing behaviors/techniques

Goals/Outcomes

- Relieve distention and excessive belching
- Reduce physical and psychological distress

Documentation in the Medical Record

Initial Medical and Psychosocial Assessment

- Potential cause(s) of eructation
- Physical examination findings (cranial nerves, swallowing, oropharynx, abdomen)
- Amount of distress/discomfort caused by symptoms
- Remedies tried by patient/caregiver with degree of success

Interdisciplinary Progress Notes

- Results of selected interventions and ongoing assessments

IDT Care Plan

- Interventions and contingency plans

Recommended Reading

Hemmink GJ, Ten Cate L, Bredenoord AJ, Timmer R, Weusten BL, Smout AJ. Speech therapy in patients with excessive supragastric belching—a pilot study. Neurogastroenterology & Motility. 2010;22(1):24–28

Hemmink GJ, Bredenoord AJ, Weusten BL, Timmer R, Smout AJ. Supragastric belching in patients with reflux symptoms. Am J Gastroenterol. 2009;104(8):1992–1997

Montalto M, Di Stefano M, Gasbarrini A, Corazza GR. Intestinal gas metabolism. Digestive and Liver Disease. 2009;3(2):27–29

Bleeding, Oozing, and Malodorous Lesions

SITUATIONS:

- Bleeding: minor, **moderate, or major** bleeding leading to distress, fatigue (anemia), excessive caregiver burden are examples .
- Malodorous lesions, exudates, drainage, etc.: these problems represent great social and emotional distress for patients and their caregivers. Not only are these conditions a constant reminder of progression of disease, but even the most loving family members and caregivers may find it difficult to stay in close contact with the patient when smells from infected or necrotic tissues and the like can be so overwhelming. Similarly, patients will feel humiliated, undignified, isolated, and often "unlovable." Thus, it is not surprising that malodor has been found to be the symptom that causes the most distress in patients who experience it, and this contributes significantly to total pain and suffering. This type of situation most flagrantly adds insult to injury, and all that can be done should be done to diminish the burden of sensory insults that drive a wedge between patient and caregivers/loved ones.

Causes

- Necrotic tissue due to tumor or ischemia
- Erosion of vascular supply by tumor
- Breakdown in skin integrity
- Infection
- Gastrointestinal disease: gastritis, peptic ulcers, inflammatory bowel disease, tumor, varices
- Nonhealing wounds due to inadequate blood supply or catabolic state
- Bleeding diathesis/coagulopathy, hematologic cancers

Findings

Biomedical

- Malodorous and oozing lesions, which can be fungating or ulcerating, drainage sites
  - Can cause fatigue, interrupted sleep patterns, anorexia, nausea, dyspnea, pruritus, lymphedema, reduced mobility and activity levels

- Can lead to signs of infection in chronic wounds, including cellulitis, malodor, pain, delayed healing, deterioration or breakdown, and increased exudates
- Can cause pain: inflammatory, neuropathic, or mixed (see "Pain" later in this section)
- 5% to 10% of patients with cancer develop a malignant wound:
  — More common in cancers from breast, gastrointestinal system, lung, head and neck, primary skin, genitourinary and gynecological sites
  — Main anatomic locations include breast and chest wall, head and neck, back, trunk, abdomen, groin, axilla, genitals
- Minor bleeding
  - Minor recurrent nosebleeds (epistaxis) or gingival bleeding caused by drying of mucous membranes or increased systolic blood pressure
  - Capillary oozing or other minor bleeding from open sores, decubiti, stomas, hemorrhoids, macerated/abraded skin (e.g., perineum)
  - Petechial bleeding as a result of thrombocytopenia
- Moderate to major bleeding
  - Gastrointestinal blood loss (melena, hematochezia, hematemesis)
  - Pulmonary blood loss (hemoptysis)
  - More vigorous blood loss from epistaxis, skin lesions, stomas, etc., as above
- Disruption of major blood vessel(s) by necrosis or tumor
- Fatigue, dyspnea, tachycardia, hypotension
- Pain may be associated with bleeding, oozing, infected, necrotic lesions
- Nausea, vomiting, diarrhea may be associated with swallowed blood or gastrointestinal bleeding

Psychosocial/Spiritual

- Many feelings are experienced and words are used by patients and family members to express what is happening, overtly and subliminally; a list of what should be explored includes:
  - Fear
  - Embarrassment
  - Disgust
  - Shame
  - Isolation
  - Guilt
  - Avoidance
  - Stigmatization
  - Depression
  - Loss of confidence
  - Anxiety
  - Worthlessness
  - Panic
  - Demoralization

Evaluation

Biomedical

- Determine source and cause of unpleasant bodily odors and drainage
- Minor bleeding
  - Determine source of bleeding.
  - Inspect open wounds and dressings for evidence of bloody drainage.
  - Determine rate/amount of bleeding.
  - Examine to identify specific bleeding site, if possible.
- Moderate to major bleeding
  - Determine likelihood of massive hemorrhagic (exsanguinating) bleed.
  - Determine site, cause, and volume of active blood loss, if possible.
- Determine relationship between signs and symptoms of fatigue with degree of anemia induced by blood loss
- Determine patient and caregiver goals of care in relation to bleeding, anemia, transfusions

NOTE: Check hematocrit only if infusion of blood products is an appropriate palliative measure in the whole context of the patient's circumstances, preferences, and goals and if bleeding site has been controlled adequately to prevent immediate loss of transfused red cells.

- Determine caregiver knowledge and ability to manage wound care and dressing changes

Psychosocial/Spiritual

- Assess emotional effect of malodorous or oozing lesions and bleeding on patient/caregiver
- Review or initiate discussions regarding advance directives in the face of massive blood loss
- Identify any specific injunctions against the use of blood products

Practical

- Identify readily accessible resources to deal with massive blood loss (e.g., dark towels, etc.)

Processes of Care

Biomedical

- Malodorous and oozing lesions: The primary approach to wound care is cleansing with sterile saline; use of peroxide or iodine-containing solutions should be reserved for cases where there is infection or necrotic tissue so that granulation is not inhibited; necrotic tissue may require active débridement, progressing from wet-to-dry dressings, to Xerogel or similar dressings, to application of enzymatic agents (e.g., streptokinase)
- Management of malodorous lesions includes an interdisciplinary team approach that can include nursing (basic or wound care specialist care) and

medical interventions, surgery, palliative radiotherapy, chemotherapy or hormonal manipulation; basic care includes:

1. Cleanse wound gently with warm normal saline and keep the wound moist.
2. Manage distressing symptoms with emphasis on comfort, appearance, odor control dressing wear times and proper fit. Anticipate bleeding. Gear efforts to stabilizing wound and preventing further deterioration.
3. Use of wound care products such as polyurethane foam and non-adhesive gel dressings to reduce pain and control exudates. Preferentially arrange for dressing choices that have a non-adherent contact layer (soft silicon perforated sheet) for exudates to be absorbed and moisture evaporated from the second layer, or alginates with a secondary retention layer of foam, and include the patient in choosing the product for comfort and longevity of wear.
   a. Activated charcoal dressings for odor control
   b. Antimicrobial dressings for infected, malodorous wounds
   c. For antisepsis, silver-impregnated dressings or cadexomer iodine are less damaging to tissues
   d. Consider metronidazole topically (0.75% or 0.8% gel or cream or 500-mg tablets crushed and sprinkled on wound bid) and/or systemically, if tolerated (500 mg PO tid) for increased odor control
4. Consider use of medical-grade irradiated, sterile, antimicrobial honey (several available brands).

- Painful cutaneous lesions (see "Pain" later in this section):
  1. Nonsteroidal anti-inflammatories (NSAIDs) are often helpful, such as ibuprofen 10 mg/kg PO tid (maximum 2,400 mg/day).
  2. Topical therapy can reduce burning and stinging (e.g., aerosolized 0.5% bupivacaine or a paste of aluminum hydroxide-magnesium hydroxide).
  3. Consider use of topical morphine (there are no commercially available products, and due to unpredictable absorption, a compounded preparation providing an initial measured "dose" of 10 mg per application, titrated to effect, is recommended).

- Minor bleeding: epistaxis
  1. Avoid disruption of crusted scabs in nose.
  2. Keep patient in high-Fowler position with head slightly bent forward.
  3. Provide constant pressure to outer nares for 5 to 10 minutes.
  4. Apply cold compresses to nape of neck.
  5. Provide cool mist humidification to room air to reduce drying of nasal passages.
  6. Provide humidification of prescribed nasal oxygen if bleeding occurs from dry nasal passages.
  7. Neo-Synephrine nasal spray up to qid: DO NOT blow nose after spray

- Minor bleeding: topical sites
  1. Obtain medical orders and instruct caregiver in use of coagulant products, as indicated:
     a. Gelfoam sponge or powder to bleeding site. Follow package directions: (1) Moisten Gelfoam sponge with sterile normal saline. (2) Apply damp sponge to bleeding wound with moderate pressure until hemostasis results. (3) Sponge may be left in place at the site, where it will dissolve, or fresh pieces may be used as needed.
     b. Silver nitrate sticks topically to bleeding site if well localized; hold stick to bleeding point followed by a gentle rotating motion.
     c. Topical sucralfate applied 1 to 2 grams crushed with water-soluble gel. Apply one or two times daily.
- Moderate to major bleeding:
  1. Prepare a "hemorrhage kit" with dressings, emergency medications, basin, dark towels, blue absorbent pads (Chux), latex gloves, washcloths, trash bags, etc., and keep kit under or near bed for any potential massive hemorrhage.
     a. To use topically applied epinephrine, dilute 1:1,000 (1 mg in 1 ml). Apply with pressure for 10 minutes; rebound bleeding may recur when effect wears off. Use with caution: it is a potent vasoconstrictor that may aggravate necrosis.
  2. Notify physician of frank bleeding episode.

NOTE: Where routine topical approaches such as pressure, epinephrine-soaked gauze, Gelfoam, and similar treatments are unsuccessful, not tolerated, or impractical, yet bleeding is continuous and profuse enough to cause distress, pharmacotherapy using fibrinolytic inhibitors may be indicated, per preferences and goals of the patient.

     a. Tranexamic acid: 1.5 g PO loading dose followed by 1 g PO tid; can also mix 500 mg in 5 ml of saline and soak into gauze, apply with pressure for 10 minutes
     b. Aminocaproic acid: 5 g PO loading dose followed by 1 g PO qid

  3. Apply pressure to bleeding site if appropriate.
  4. Change saturated dressings as needed.
  5. Camouflage obvious blood loss if possible.
  6. Use dark-colored towels to absorb blood.
  7. Cover urinary drainage bag in presence of gross hematuria.
  8. Remove soiled dressings or bedclothes as soon as possible.
  9. Irrigate Foley catheter with normal saline to maintain patency if urinary bleeding.
  10. Instruct caregiver(s) on universal precautions and handling of bodily fluids (see "Basic Home Safety" in Section Two).
  11. Obtain orders for anxiolytic medications (see "Agitation and Anxiety" earlier in this section). Diazepam injectable for IM use may be the most expedient approach if the patient is experiencing significant emotional distress with potentially fatal bleeding. Can also use lorazepam 4 mg

sublingual (rate of onset 5 minutes) or diazepam 10 suppository (rate of onset 10 to 15 minutes) if IM diazepam is unavailable or the caregiver is unable to use the IM route due to his or her own anxiety with injection.

12. Consider use of palliative radiotherapy in selected cases, in anticipation of potential for bleeding, or after initial bleed is controlled, if consistent with life expectancy and goals of care.

Psychosocial

- Identify patients potentially at risk: site of cancer (i.e., head and neck, hematologic), presentation with bleeding (i.e., hemoptysis), coexisting disease predisposing patient to bleed (e.g., GI bleeding, liver failure, esophageal varices), smaller warning bleeding, local infection at tumor site, clotting abnormalities, or use of drugs predisposing patient to bleeding, such as heparin, coumadin, or enoxaparin
- Explain what to expect if bleeding does occur and explain purpose of "hemorrhage kit"
- Inform caregiver that bleeding episodes may be accompanied by symptoms of anxiety, restlessness, cool moist skin, and increased pallor
- Instruct caregiver to call hospice nurse or extended coverage staff if hemorrhage should occur
- In the event of brisk bleeding, stay with patient/caregiver
- Initiate continuous care until bleeding is controlled or stops
- Explain option to transfer patient to a contracted facility if the caregiver or patient is extremely anxious and unlikely to cope with impending situation

Goals/Outcomes

- Minimize emotional distress and social isolation
- Reduce or stop bleeding from all sites to the extent possible
- Maintain patient's red cell mass/oxygen-carrying capacity in order to prevent anemia-related fatigue and to avoid or minimize the need for palliative red cell transfusion
- Prevent caregiver avoidance of patient
- Facilitate reasoned self-determination about various approaches to therapy for symptomatic blood loss, especially in the consideration of palliative transfusion
- Prevent panic in the event of frank hemorrhage

Documentation in the Medical Record

Initial Medical and Psychosocial Assessment

- Causes and severity of malodorous lesions/sources and bleeding
- Patient/caregiver reaction(s) to malodorous lesions/sources and bleeding
- Likelihood of hemorrhagic event
- Symptoms/signs of anemia

Interdisciplinary Progress Notes

- Content of discussions and results of interventions

- Results of ongoing assessments

IDT Care Plan

- Proposed interventions and contingency plans
- Schedule of reassessments

Recommended Reading

Alexander S. Malignant fungating wounds: epidemiology, aetiology, presentation and assessment. J Wound Care. 2009;18(7):273–280

Alexander S. Malignant fungating wounds: key symptoms and psychosocial issues. J Wound Care. 2009;18(8):325–329

Cartoni C, Niscola P, Breccia M, et al. Hemorrhagic complications in patients with advanced hematological malignancies followed at home: an Italian experience. Leukemia Lymphoma. 2009;50(3):387–391

Chrisman C. Care of chronic wounds in palliative care and end-of-life patients. Intl Wound J. 2010;7(4):214–235

Da Costo Santos C, Pimenta C, Nobre MA. Systematic review of topical treatments to control the odor of malignant fungating wounds. J Pain Symptom Management. 2010;39(6):1065–1076

Hulme B, Wilcox S. Guidelines on the management of bleeding for palliative care patients with cancer. Yorkshire Palliative Medicine Clinical Guidelines Group. November 2008. see www.palliativedrugs.com/download/090331_Final_bleeding_guidelines.pdf

LaBon B, Zeppetella G Higginson I. Effectiveness of topical administration of opioids in palliative care: A systematic review. J Pain Symptom Management. 2009;37(5):913–917

Lipsky B, Hoey C. Topical antimicrobial therapy for treating chronic wounds. Clinical Infectious Dis. 2009;49:1541–1549

Merz T, Klein C, Uebach B, Kern M, Ostgathe C, Bukki J. Fungating wounds—multidimensional challenge in palliative care. J Breast Care. 2011;6(1):21–24

Patel B, Cox-Hayley D. Managing wound odor. J Palliative Med. 2010;13(10):1286–1287

Confusion/Delirium

SITUATION: Change in mental status with acute confusion that interferes with ability to carry out activities of daily living, patient safety, and adds to caregiver burden

Causes

Biomedical

- Systemic infection (e.g., common occurrence in the elderly with urinary tract infection, pneumonia)
- Dehydration
- Toxic drug reactions (e.g., anticholinergic effects from scopolamine, tricyclic antidepressants, anxiolytics, corticosteroids, antiemetics, sedatives)

- Organic brain syndrome from underlying disease (e.g., AIDS dementia, hydro-cephalus, degenerative brain changes, neoplasm, cerebrovascular occlusion or bleeding)
- Metabolic or physiologic derangement (e.g., hypercalcemia, hyponatremia, hyper/hypoglycemia, electrolyte imbalance, uremia, thyroid dysfunction, adrenal disease, advanced liver, renal, or respiratory impairment, fecal impaction, urinary retention
- Acute abstinence syndrome (alcohol, opioids, benzodiazepines, psychoactive drugs)

Psychosocial/Spiritual

- Psychological decompensation from social stressors
- Depression ("pseudo-dementia")
- Fear
- Anxiety
- Pathological grief reaction in anticipation of loss
- Environmental
  - Hospitalization/ICU disorientation
  - Sleep deprivation
  - Psychological stress from noxious procedures (e.g., urethral catheterization)
  - Communication impairment

Findings

Biomedical

- Stigmata of coexisting disease to be found during systemic review and physical examination
- Decreased or increased level of activity (i.e., somnolent versus restless/agitated)

Psychosocial

- Alterations in perception and cognition (i.e., decreased or fluctuating level of consciousness, disorientation, and misperception); may become evident only after a long discussion or several visits with the patient

Evaluation

Biomedical

- Review medications for drugs that may cause or contribute to confusion, especially recently added psychotropic agents or changes in drug or dosing schedule
- Collect data from family or caregivers regarding patient's mental status before the onset of delirium
- Assess for metabolic derangement based on likelihoods (e.g., blood sugar abnormalities in a known diabetic)
- Associated signs and symptoms
  - Uremia: oliguria/anuria; "frost" on facial skin

- Hyperglycemia: polydipsia, polyuria, blurred vision, "fruity" odor to breath
- Hypoglycemia: lethargy to unarousability, tachycardia, diaphoresis
- Hypercalcemia: polydipsia, polyuria, nausea, ileus, muscle twitching
- Determine relative burdens (intrusiveness and costs of tests) versus benefits (likelihood of improvement from specific therapeutic interventions) in concert with patient/family goals
- Assess for presence of fever or common sources of infection: urinary, respiratory, skin (pressure sores, abscess, cellulitis)
- Assess for signs of neurologic change to suggest brain metastasis:
  - Volatile mood/behavior or fluctuating level of consciousness, hallucinations, thought disorder
  - Headache
  - Nausea/vomiting
  - Visual impairment (double vision; field cut)
  - Motor, sensory, coordination alteration or deficit
  - Papilledema
- Assess for withdrawal symptoms from alcohol or other drugs:
  - Time of last dose or drink
  - Tachycardia, tachypnea, diaphoresis, hypertension
  - Nausea, abdominal pain, diarrhea
  - Pupillary dilatation (mydriasis)
  - Restlessness, hallucinosis, paranoia

Psychosocial

- Perform Mini-Mental Status Examination (compare with previous baseline if available):
  - Orientation (person, place, time, situation)
  - Remote and recent memory (last four presidents, children's/grandchildren's names/birthdates, ability to recall four items after 5 to 10 minutes)
  - Cognitive function (ability to read simple text and comprehend it; ability to subtract serial 7s from 100; ability to tell time)
  - Reasoning (what would you do if you smelled smoke in the house?)
  - Abstraction (what does "people who live in glass houses shouldn't throw stones" mean?)
  - Spatial integrity (draw a round clock face with numbers and hands)
  - Assess for presence of insomnia
  - Assess for presence of delusions and/or hallucinations
- Other assessment tools include Confusion Assessment Method (CAM; see http://consultgerirn.org/uploads/File/trythis/try_this_13.pdf) and Memorial Delirium Assessment Scale (MDAS; see http://crashingpatient.com/wp-content/pdf/MDAS.pdf)

Processes of Care

Practical

- Instruct caregiver(s) on reality orientation (frequent reminders of time and place; provide cues such as large-numbered calendar and clock)
- Allay fear: use visual and hearing aids
- Instruct caregiver(s) on need for simple, structured routine and quiet, calm environment as much as possible
- Provide interventions to ensure adequate periods of rest
- "Routine-ize" defecation/urination (for continent patients), nutrition, mobilization

Biomedical

- Medicate according to need for patient safety, to relieve distressing symptoms and to obtain reasonable periods of rest, per physician orders
- Notify attending physician if assessment indicates an etiology that is new or imminently treatable
- Pharmacotherapy for palliation of delirium/agitation unrelieved by primary therapies or milieu therapy. Note: no medications have been approved by the U.S. Food and Drug Administration (FDA) with specific indications for the treatment of delirium
  1. Haloperidol 0.5 to 1.0 mg PO q6hr; titrate upward as needed.
  2. Lorazepam may be added to haloperidol in severe agitation and dangerous behavior related to delirium. Lorazepam alone is ineffective in the treatment of delirium.
  3. Chlorpromazine is an acceptable alternative (25 mg PO/PR q6–8hr) to haloperidol if greater sedation is desirable.
  4. Atypical antipsychotics (risperidone 0.5 to 1 mg bid, olanzapine 2.5 to 5 mg/day, quetiapine 50 to 100 mg bid) are alternatives in managing delirium. The FDA has issued a black box warning of increased risk of death when these antipsychotics are used to treat elderly patients with dementia-related psychoses.
  5. Follow guidelines in "Agitation and Anxiety" earlier in this section if confusional state progresses to a more severe state of agitation.

Psychosocial

- Provide a quiet environment: reduce unnecessary noise, activity, clutter
- Speak clearly in simple short sentences; avoid complex explanations; be sure patient can hear you
- Direct patient's attention on the present
- Identify and focus on patient's strengths
- Involve social worker early to assist patient and caregiver with coping skills and to identify need for volunteers and other expertise within the IDT
- Provide support to caregiver
  - Anticipate cognitive changes with disease progression and educate caregivers to report early, potentially reversible alternations in mental status.

- Believe caregiver's observations about changes in patient's mental state (these may be subtle to outside observers who see the patient on an occasional basis only).
- Arrange for volunteer to relieve family.
- Assist family to schedule rest periods so that someone is resting when another is with the patient.
- Allow caregiver to voice concerns, sadness, and/or anger regarding change in patient's personality.

Goals/Outcomes

- Patient is able to rest comfortably without excessive fear, agitation, or restlessness
- Maximize patient's ability to communicate needs and express feelings
- Caregiver burden is minimized to allow adequate periods of rest, sleep, and uninterrupted household activities
- Safe environment is provided for patient and caregiver
- Prevent unnecessary transfers

Documentation in the Medical Record

Initial Medical Assessment

- Precipitating factors leading to confusion
- Signs and symptoms of concurrent or progressive disease
- Findings from systems review and physical examination
- Differential diagnosis of etiology of acute signs/symptoms

Initial Psychosocial Assessment

- Patient behaviors and results of mental status examination
- Goals of therapy and advance directives reviewed/discussed

Interdisciplinary Progress Notes

- Results of interventions
- Observations from repeated assessments
- Caregiver coping

IDT Care Plan

- Order of evaluation and treatment approaches
- Specific interventions
- Contingency plans

Recommended Reading

Abrahm JL. Advances in palliative medicine and end-of-life care. Ann Rev Med. 2011;62:187–199

Breitbart W, Alici Y. Agitation and delirium at the end of life. JAMA. 2008;300(24):2898–2910 Moyer DD. Terminal delirium in geriatric patients with cancer at end of life. Am J Hospice Palliative Med. 2011;28(1):44–51

Rao S, Ferris FD, Irwin SA. Ease of screening for depression and delirium in patients enrolled in inpatient hospice care. J Palliative Med. 2011;14(3):275–279

Constipation

SITUATION: Decreased bowel motility with consequent constipation, distention, obstipation, or impaction

Causes

- Decreased autonomic function due to aging
- Decreased activity
- Alterations in food and fluid intake
- Inaccessibility of toilet due to decreased mobility, sedation, etc., leading to retention of stool
- Pharmacological effects of opioid analgesics and drugs with anticholinergic activity (e.g., tricyclic antidepressants)
- Painful anorectal lesions (e.g., hemorrhoids, fissures) leading to retention of stool
- Weakness due to primary disease or secondary to asthenia
- Hypokalemia; hypercalcemia

Findings

- Patient report or caregiver assessment of decreased bowel movement frequency, hard stool, or painful elimination
- Soiling of clothing due to seepage of liquid stool around impacted stool in rectum
- Sense of bloating with abdominal distention
- Increase or absence of bowel sounds
- No bowel movement for at least 2 days
- Painful anal lesions

Evaluation

- Bowel assessment should be a regular part of every patient visit. Consider use of a constipation assessment scale such as the Constipation Assessment Scale or the Constipation Visual Analogue Scale (see http://www.thefreelibrary.com/Modified+Constipation+Assessment+Scale+is+an+effective+tool+to+assess ... -a0138224937)
- Determine date of last bowel movement and stool characteristics
- Review 24-hour food and fluid intake
- Determine patient's ability to respond to urge to defecate (generate adequate bearing down)
- Determine patient's ability to get to toilet or notify caregiver for help in toileting
- Auscultate and examine abdomen for quality and intensity (or absence) of bowel sounds, masses, and tenderness
- Observe, percuss, and palpate abdomen for distention, tympany, and tenderness

- Assess for and rule out urinary retention commonly associated with fecal impaction
- Determine if new-onset nausea/vomiting is present, suspicious for bowel obstruction
- Perform an anorectal examination for lesions, muscle tone, retained stool, impaction

Processes of Care

Practical and Biomedical

- Notify physician if evidence of bowel obstruction
- Convenience (access to facilities), comfort, and privacy (dignity) should be optimized to promote regular bowel movements and prevent retention
- All patients taking opioid analgesics should be on some form of anticonstipation regimen
- Increase hydration if consistent with patient wishes and benefits would likely outweigh burdens
- Never use motility agents when there are signs or symptoms of bowel obstruction
- Disimpaction and enemas should precede use of motility agents
- Recommend or allow use of psyllium (e.g., Metamucil) or bulking foods and fiber (fruits, bran, etc.) in active and well-hydrated patients only
- Pharmacotherapy for constipation
  - Rectal suppositories should be placed up against wall of the rectum, not in substance of stool
  - Glycerin suppositories for dry, hard, difficult-to-pass stool
  - Starting anticonstipation regimen
    — Senna preparation (e.g., Senokot tabs one or two tabs PO q HS, and increase up to four tabs tid [may substitute 5 ml of liquid Senokot for each tablet]) as needed; or
    — Bisacodyl 5 mg, one or two tablets PO at HS or bisacodyl 10-mg suppository PR at HS); double, then triple the dose, adding morning and afternoon doses
  - If no bowel movement within 24 to 48 hours, for hard, desiccated stool, add a stool softener (e.g., docusate sodium 250 mg qd to bid)
  - If no bowel movement within 48 hours of initiating therapy, use phosphate (Fleet) enema
- If no bowel movement within 72 hours of initiating therapy, repeat rectal examination; if no evidence of bowel obstruction, no impaction, and no result from oil retention enema (4 oz warmed mineral oil or Fleet Mineral Oil Enema) followed by phosphate enema:
  - Magnesium citrate 8 oz PO or mineral oil 30 to 60 ml PO
  - Lactulose 10 to 30 ml PO qd or bid
- Peripheral opioid antagonist therapy
  - Methylnaltrexone is a peripherally acting mu-opioid receptor antagonist with restricted ability to cross the blood–brain barrier; it reverses opioid-induced constipation without affecting analgesia\

- The recommended dose of the approved injectable form of methylnaltrexone is 8 mg for patients weighing 38 to 62 kg (84 to 136 lb) or 12 mg for patients weighing 62 to 114 kg (136 to 251 lb); patients whose weight falls outside of these ranges should be dosed at 0.15 mg/kg
- Studies have reported that between 48% and 62% of patients treated with methylnaltrexone have a bowel movement within 4 hours of subcutaneous administration; ensure that there is no impaction before administration
- Manual disimpaction
  - Apply local anesthetic preparation (e.g., eutectic mixture of local anesthetic [EMLA cream], lidocaine 2% ointment or 4% gel) liberally to external and internal anal mucosa and administer 4 oz of warm mineral oil into rectal vault 15 to 30 minutes prior to digital dilatation and stool removal
  - If this process causes distress, especially when repeat disimpaction is required, premedication with lorazepam 1 to 2 mg and the patient's usual breakthrough dose of analgesic 30 to 60 minutes before manual disimpaction will usually produce favorable conditions

Goals/Outcomes

- Painless, regular bowel movements at least every 3 days
- Absence of induced diarrhea and abdominal cramping from bowel regimen
- Confidence in use of opioid analgesics for pain relief without worry over bowel function

Documentation in the Medical Record

Admission Assessment

- Review of bowel function
- Risks of impending bowel dysfunction due to disease, medications, activity, food/fluid intake
- Patient's and/or family caregiver's ability to manage own bowel care
- Physical examination findings
- Medication review
- Dietary assessment

Interdisciplinary Progress Notes

- History of bowel actions and toileting ability
- Use of bowel protocol
- Therapeutic and adverse effects of bowel protocol
- Findings from repeated physical examination

IDT Care Plan

- Progressive implementation of bowel protocol
- Instructions to patient/caregiver
- Schedule of follow-up evaluations of adherence to bowel protocol and reassessments

Recommended Reading

Chamberlain BH, Cross K, Winston JL, et al. Methylnaltrexone treatment of opioid-induced constipation in patients with advanced illness. J Pain Symptom Manage. 2009;38(5):683–690

Goodman M, Low J, Wilkinson S. Constipation management in palliative care: a survey of practices in the United Kingdom. J Pain Symptom Manage. 2005;29:238–244

Larkin PJ, Sykes NP, Centeno C, Ellershaw JE, et al; European Consensus Group on Constipation in Palliative Care. Palliat Med. 2008;22(7):796–807

Slatkin N, Thomas J, Lipman AG, et al. Methylnaltrexone for treatment of opioid-induced constipation in advanced illness patients. J Support Oncol. 2009;7(1):39–46

Thomas J, Karver S, Cooney GA, et al. Methylnaltrexone for opioid-induced constipation in advanced illness. N Engl J Med. 2008;358(22):2332–2343

Coughing

SITUATION: Frequent cough with resultant pain or discomfort, inability to rest, social disruption, and interruption of sleep

Causes

- Pulmonary infection
- COPD
- Decreased mobility
- Weakness with reduced effectiveness of cough (ineffective clearing of airways)
- Sinus infection
- Respiratory system neoplasm
- Pulmonary edema
- Pleural effusion
- Reactive airways disease (asthma)

Findings

- Loose, productive cough
- Dry, nonproductive cough
- Exasperation, exhaustion, chest pain

Evaluation

Biomedical

- History of new-onset versus recurrent versus chronic cough
- Review history of smoking, asthma, occupational factors
- Obtain history of triggering and relieving factors
- Assess cough (frequency, quality, intensity, muscle power)
- Assess sputum characteristics (volume, color, purulence)

- Auscultate lungs for adventitious breath sounds (rhonchi, rales, wheezes), diminished breath sounds, pleural rub
- Check for peripheral edema, jugular venous distention, gallop rhythm
- Rule out associated paroxysmal nocturnal dyspnea or orthopnea
- Check for use of accessory muscles of respiration, tachypnea, tachycardia, cyanosis
- Assess for fever
- Check for sinus tenderness, nasal discharge

Psychosocial

- Assess impact of cough on mood, sleep, energy, pain, social interaction

Processes of Care

Biomedical

- Treat specific etiology of cough if identified (e.g., antibiotics, diuretics, bronchodilators)
- Instruct in proper use of nebulizer, if indicated
- Aggressively treat symptoms in concert with the degree of distress being caused
- Increase humidity in patient's environment—cool mist vaporizer in room
- Elevate head (of bed)
- Palliative pharmacotherapy
  a. Guaifenesin 5 ml PO q4hr prn or one or two tablets PO q12hr up to four tablets/24 hr
  b. Dextromethorphan-containing cough syrup: use as directed (usually 1 to 2 tsp PO q4hr)
  c. Codeine 15 to 30 mg PO q4hr prn

NOTE: Adjust dose based on other opioid analgesic use and institute constipation prevention/treatment care plan.

  d. Treat insomnia if nocturnal cough unabated by above therapies (refer to "Insomnia and Nocturnal Restlessness" later in this section)
  e. Nebulized opioids and local anesthetics
    - Opioid receptors are expressed in bronchopulmonary tissues with great variability
    - Consider nebulized opioids or lidocaine in severe, refractory cases (data mixed on efficacy, no high-quality data exist)
    - Initial opioid dosing: morphine 5 mg/2 ml in 0.9% saline or fentanyl 25 mcg/2 ml in saline (fentanyl, being more lipophilic and less allergenic, may be advantageous)
    - Initial local anesthetic dosing: lidocaine 5 ml of 2% solution (cautious titration and frequency of dosing due to variable absorption and risk of systemic toxicity)
- Instruct in appropriate handling and disposal of sputum (refer to "Basic Home Safety" in Section Two)

Goals/Outcomes

- Ability to clear airways and expectorate sputum and bronchopulmonary secretions
- Reduce coughing paroxysms to the extent possible based on the underlying disease
- Increase periods of rest and uninterrupted sleep
- Improve social interaction
- Maximize hygiene
- Prevent and treat cough-related pain

Documentation in the Medical Record

Initial Assessment

- Findings of cardiopulmonary systems review and physical examination
- Impact of cough on patient/caregiver

Interdisciplinary Progress Notes

- Results of interventions and ongoing assessments

IDT Care Plan

- Specific interventions and associated goals
- Follow-up and contingency plans

Recommended Reading

Ben-Aharon I, Gafter-Gvili A, Paul M. Interventions for alleviating cancer-related dyspnea: a systematic review. J Clin Oncol. 2008;26:2396–2404

Hayes D, Anstead M, Warner R, Kuhn R, Ballard H. Inhaled morphine for palliation of dyspnea in end-stage cystic fibrosis. Am J Health-System Pharmacy. 2010;67(9):737–740

Lingerfelt BM, Swainey CW, Smith TJ, Coyne PJ. Nebulized lidocaine for intractable cough near the end of life. J Support Oncol. 2007;5(7):301–302

Molassiotis A, Smith J, Bennett M, et al. Clinical expert guidelines for the management of cough in lung cancer: report of a UK task group on cough. Cough. 2010;6:9

Wee B. Chronic cough. Curr Opin Support Palliat Care. 2008;2(2):105–109

Zu-ming Lv, Li C, Jie Tang. Nebulized lidocaine inhalation in the treatment of patients with acute asthma. World J Emerg Med. 2011;2(1):30–32

Depression

SITUATION: Depressed mood that interferes with patient care or patient/caregiver ability to cope with the dying process

Causes

Biomedical

- Primary affective disorder
- Unrelieved pain

- Uncontrolled distressing symptoms
- Sleep disorder
- Underlying primary disease-related mood disturbance
- Adverse effect of certain medications (e.g., antihypertensive therapy)

Psychosocial/Spiritual

- Anticipatory grief reaction
- Response to actual loss: function, self-image, future, crisis of faith, etc.
- Boredom, social isolation, sense of uselessness/purposelessness/meaninglessness, lack of goals

Findings

Biomedical

- Sleep disturbance
- Uncontrolled pain or other distressing symptoms (e.g., nausea, chronic cough, etc.)
- Vegetative or agitated behaviors
- Inappropriate medication/substance use or frank misuse of mood-altering agents (alcohol, psychotropic drugs, analgesics, sedative-hypnotics)

Psychosocial/Spiritual

- Verbal or facial expression of low mood, sadness
- Flat affect, crying, social withdrawal, isolation
- "Vegetative signs" (e.g., hypersomnolence, decreased appetite, psychomotor retardation, anhedonia)
- Occasional agitation, volatility, flares of anger
- Self-deprecation, guilt, hopelessness, self-recrimination

Evaluation

Biomedical

- Determine role of underlying disease or uncontrolled symptoms as cause of depression
- Evaluate effect of medications on signs and symptoms of depression

Psychosocial/Spiritual

- Directly ask the question: "Are you depressed?" and rate the response using 0-to-5 scale
- Review of past psychiatric history and response to loss or difficult life events
- Understand patient/caregiver's perception of situation
- Differentiate symptoms as a reaction to circumstances from primary affective disorder, if possible: refer to *DSM-IV-TR*
- Identify patient/caregiver's understanding of, and capacity to address, depression
- Assess severity of depression and likelihood of suicide (refer to "Suicide: Risk, Prevention, Coping When It Happens" in Section Two)

- Assess impact of depression on care and ability to cope
- Facilitate discussion surrounding faith, values, definitions of hope and meaningfulness to determine potential role of spiritual crisis on depressed mood

Processes of Care

Biomedical

- Consult with physician regarding possible contributory medications and adjustments
- Discuss indications for antidepressant pharmacotherapy during IDT review
- Pharmacotherapy for treatment of depression:

NOTE: Supportive counseling and empathic listening by members of the IDT (RN, social worker, chaplain, aide[s], physician, volunteers) should complement pharmacotherapy. Selection of antidepressant medications should be based on symptoms, safety, simplicity of dosing, rapidity of response based on prognosis, safety profile, burden of adverse/side effects, and cost.

1. Depression associated with significant sleep disturbance:
   a. Trazodone 50 mg PO HS, titrated up by 50-mg increments as tolerated q3–5days to 400 mg; monitor closely for efficacy versus adverse effects (e.g., excessive daytime sedation)
   b. Sedating tricyclic antidepressants (e.g., amitriptyline, doxepin) are effective alternatives for sleep disturbance, but anticholinergic effects are more problematic, especially with dose escalation to antidepressant levels; combined use with an SSRI antidepressant (see below) is recommended; monitor for metabolic disturbances and drug–drug interactions that can lead to central serotonin toxicity
   c. Mirtazapine 15 mg PO HS, titrated up by 15-mg increments as tolerated every week up to 45 mg

NOTE: A therapeutic antidepressant effect may take several weeks, but improvements in sleep should occur rapidly, especially at lower doses.

1. Depression without significant sleep disturbance:
   a. Psychostimulants (e.g., methylphenidate 2.5 to 10 mg PO every morning and mid-day) for management of acute depression, especially with very limited life expectancy
   b. Paroxetine 20 mg PO every morning (10 mg every morning in frail, elderly patients), or
   c. Fluoxetine 20 mg PO every morning, or
   d. Sertraline 50 mg PO every morning, or
   e. Venlafaxine 25 mg PO tid

Psychosocial/Practical/Spiritual

- Initiate discussion and promote expression of thoughts and feelings
- Facilitate discussion of losses
- Identify and reflect distortions in thinking
- Help patient/caregiver understand and accept limits imposed by illness and assuage frustration of trying to control the uncontrollable

- Help patient/caregiver identify what areas in their lives are still under their control
- Help identify attainable goals
- Engage patient/caregiver in life review
- Identify and facilitate social interactions and recreational/distracting activities that may give meaning to daily life
- Determine if any foods give pleasure, regardless of nutritional value, and make available if possible
- Determine patient's need to search for meaning in the dying experience and help him/her to find the language to express this
- Understand patient's values and preferences and facilitate these choices during the dying process to the extent possible
- Help patient/caregiver to identify and use positive coping skills
- Seek out and defer to expert medical/psychiatric treatment if signs/symptoms of depression do not respond to first-line approaches or if risk of suicide is high

Goals/Outcomes

- Reduce "vegetative" signs and symptoms
- Patient/caregiver will be able to openly express feelings of loss
- Patient/caregiver will identify strategies to address depression
- Patient/caregiver will report improved sense of well-being and ability to cope
- The processes of life review and addressing issues raised by the level of debility and realizations imposed by progressive disease and foreseeable death will allow the opportunity for personal growth and finding value in the remaining days of life

Documentation in the Medical Record

Initial Assessment

- Description of mood, sleep, activity, patient short-term goals (if any), patient's identified reasons for low mood
- Patient's self-rating of depression (e.g., 0-to-5 scale: 0 = "Good mood; I do not feel sad or depressed at all" and 5 = "My mood is as low as it could possibly be. I find no meaning in my life.")

Interdisciplinary Team Notes

- Description of interventions and results
- Repeat patient self-reports of depression scores (0-to-5 scale).
- Patient short-term (daily/weekly) attainable goals and results

IDT Care Plan

- Interventions planned
- Means to help patient attain stated goals
- Schedule of IDT visits

Recommended Reading

Candy B, Jones L, Williams R, Tookman A, King M. Psychostimulants for depression. Cochrane Database of Systematic Reviews. 2008; Issue 2. Art. No.: CD006722. DOI: 10.1002/14651858.CD006722.pub2. see: http://onlinelibrary.wiley.com/o/cochrane/clsysrev/articles/CD006722/frame.html

Holman A, Leurent B, Davis S, Jones L. Hospice care delivered at home, in nursing homes and in dedicated hospice facilities: A systematic review of quantitative and qualitative evidence. Int J Nurs Stud. 2011;48(1):121–33

Gelenberg AJ. Using assessment tools to screen for, diagnose, and treat major depressive disorder in clinical practice. J Clin Psychiatry. 2010;71[Suppl E1]:e01

Institute for Clinical Systems Improvement. Health Care Guideline: Major Depression in Adults in Primary Care, 11th ed., May 2008

Katon W, Lin EHB, Kroenke K. The association of depression and anxiety with medical symptom burden in patients with chronic medical illness. General Hospital Psychiatry. 2007;29(2):147–155

Mottram PG, Wilson K, Strobl J. Antidepressants for depressed elderly. Cochrane Database of Systematic Reviews. 2006; Issue 1. Art. No.: CD003491. DOI: 10.1002/14651858.CD003491.pub2. see: http://onlinelibrary.wiley.com/o/cochrane/clsysrev/articles/CD003491/frame.html

Unutzer J. Clinical practice. Late-life depression. N Engl J Med. 2007;357:2269–2276

Diarrhea and Anorectal Problems

SITUATION: Frequent watery or excessively loose stools with or without anorectal irritation, pain, or pruritus

Causes

- Overtreatment of constipation or adverse effect of laxative regimen
- Fecal impaction (overflow incontinence)
- Diet-related
- Drug-related (e.g., antibiotic-associated diarrhea)
- Infectious (viral, fungal, bacterial, or other consequence of immunosuppression or antibiotic treatment, including *C. difficile*)
- Partial bowel obstruction
- Carcinoid tumor
- Post-gastrectomy "dumping" syndrome
- Pancreatic insufficiency
- Post-radiation or chemotherapy syndrome
- Anorectal tumor

Findings

- Frequent liquid stool (more than three or four bowel movements in 24 hours)
- Abdominal cramping
- Hyperactive bowel sounds
- Anal pain, burning, irritation, itching, tenesmus (feeling of incomplete evacuation)

Evaluation

- Determine usual bowel habits and patterns, duration and extent of change
- Review current medications and bowel regimen (cathartics, laxatives, stool softeners)
- Review dietary intake and past history of bowel disorders
- Determine relationship between current disease process and propensity for bowel dysfunction
- Systems review for concomitant nausea/vomiting/fever/abdominal pain, blood in stool, number of bowel movements, consistency/color/odor/quality of stool (floating or greasy stool, clay-like, etc.)
- Auscultate bowel sounds and gently palpate abdomen for abnormal findings
- Visually examine perineum and anus, and perform digital examination to determine presence of fecal impaction
- General examination to determine if patient is dehydrated: tongue and mucous membranes, skin turgor, orthostatic blood pressure/pulse changes

Processes of Care

Practical and Biomedical

- General:
  a. Notify physician if new or rapidly advancing signs/symptoms (e.g., abdominal distention, suspected bowel obstruction, gastrointestinal bleeding, severe dehydration, etc.)
  b. Discontinue cathartics/laxatives until symptoms abate and then reinstitute gradually
  c. Clear fluids with slowly advancing diet as symptoms allow and appetite dictates
  d. Rehydrate orally if possible; otherwise, consider subcutaneous infusion (hypodermoclysis) of normal saline if prognosis warrants, unless absolutely necessary medications cannot be delivered by this route and intravenous access is necessary
- SQ hydration: Normal saline with 500 units/L hyaluronidase (only if readily available, to enhance absorption); infuse at 0.5 to 1.0 ml/kg/hr with a maximum rate of 60 ml/hr, using a 25-gauge butterfly needle inserted at a 45-degree angle to the skin, or a subcutaneous "button" device
  e. Nonspecific pharmacotherapy:
    — Kaopectate 60 ml q2hr until diarrhea stops, or
    — Loperamide HCl (Imodium AD) 2 to 4 mg PO after each loose stool (1 tablet = 2 mg, or 5 ml liquid formulation = 1 mg). If ineffective, try:
    — Diphenoxylate HCl (Lomotil) one or two tablets after each loose stool
- Etiology-specific approaches to therapy:
  a. Carcinoid tumors
    — Octreotide 150 to 300 µg SQ bid or q24hr by continuous infusion

b. Dumping syndrome (postgastrectomy)
   — Small low-carbohydrate meals
   — Eat slowly, chew thoroughly, and drink liquids between meals rather than with meals.
   — Octreotide 150–300 µg SQ bid or up to 750 µg q24hr by continuous infusion

c. Candidiasis (due to immunosuppression or antibiotic therapy)
   — Clotrimazole 10 to 20 mg PO tid or fluconazole 150 mg PO every morning
   — Loperamide 2 to 4 mg PO up to 16 mg/day. If ineffective, try:
   — Diphenoxylate one tablet PO after each diarrheal stool up to eight tablets per day
   — Tincture of opium (if available); otherwise, codeine elixir or oral morphine solution titrated to effect

d. Pancreatic insufficiency
   — Pancreatic enzyme replacement (with meals)
   — Famotidine 20 mg PO bid or omeprazole 20 mg daily
   — Loperamide 2 to 4 mg PO up to 16 mg/day. If ineffective, try:
   — Diphenoxylate one tablet PO after each diarrheal stool up to eight tablets per day

e. Post-radiation or chemotherapy syndrome
   — Eliminate fiber and milk products
   — NSAIDs (e.g., ibuprofen, celecoxib) to counteract inflammatory effects leading to radiation enteritis (see "Pain" later in this section) if tolerated and not contraindicated
   — Progressive trial of loperamide, diphenoxylate, tincture of opium (if available); otherwise, codeine elixir or oral morphine solution, titrated to control symptoms
   — Octreotide 100 µg SQ bid for otherwise uncontrolled chemotherapy-induced enteritis

f. Anal irritation
   — Clear warm water nonabrasive cleansing and thorough drying
   — Apply zinc oxide to unbroken skin
   — Apply corticosteroid cream (preparations with or without local anesthetic) to macerated or inflamed skin 1 to 2 days only

g. Rectal tumors
   — If prognosis warrants, consider palliative radiation therapy or endoscopic laser therapy
   — Hydrocortisone foam, one applicator PR bid
   — EMLA cream or other topical local anesthetic formulation prn
   — For severe pruritus ani, use a sedating antihistamine (e.g., promethazine 12.5 mg PO HS)

Goals/Outcomes

- Regular well-formed stools to the extent possible, limited only by underlying disease and patient tolerance/preference of interventions
- Ability to ingest foods of choice without undue discomfort or diarrhea
- Absence of perineal/anal discomfort

Documentation in the Medical Record

Initial Assessment

- Number and character of bowel movements
- Likely etiology of diarrhea
- Contributing factors to diarrhea
- Patient/caregiver approaches to controlling diarrhea
- Findings from physical examination

Interdisciplinary Progress Notes

- Therapies applied and results of interventions
- Findings from reassessment: frequency/quality of bowel movements and associated symptoms; physical examination

IDT Care Plan

- Interventions planned and schedule of reassessments
- Contingency plans

Recommended Reading

Abernethy A. Management of gastrointestinal symptoms in advanced cancer patients: the rapid learning cancer clinical model. Current Opinion in Supportive and Palliative Care. 2010;4(1):36–45

Bisanz A. Summary of the causative and treatment factors of diarrhea and the use of a diarrhea assessment and treatment tool to improve patient outcomes. Gastroenterology Nursing. 2010;33(4):268–281

Cherny N. Evaluation and management of treatment-related diarrhea in patients with advanced cancer: A review. J Pain Symptom Management. 2008;36(4): 413–423

Gao XW. Dose response efficacy of a proprietary probiotic formula of *Lactobacillus acidophilus cl1285* and *Lactobacillus casei LBC80R* for antibiotic-associated diarrhea and *Clostridium difficile*-associated diarrhea prophylaxis in adult patients. Am J Gastroenterol. 2010;105(7):1636–1641

Jain V. Gastrointestinal side effects of prescription medications in the older adult. J Clin Gastroenterol. 2009;43(2):103–110

Prommer E. Established and potential therapeutic applications of octreotide in palliative care. Supportive Care in Cancer. 2008;16:1117–1123

Roach M. Fecal incontinence in the elderly. Geriatrics. 2008;63(2):13–22

Zaharoni H. Probiotics improve bowel movements in hospitalized elderly patients—the PROTAGE study. J Nutrition Health Aging. 2011;15(3):215–220

Dysphagia and Oropharyngeal Problems

SITUATION: Choking with eating or drinking, difficult or painful swallowing, mucositis, oral candidiasis (thrush), and other painful or distressing/disturbing oropharyngeal conditions associated with advanced disease

Causes

- Dysphagia, with or without oral candidiasis or mucositis, commonly occurs in patients:
  a. With cancers of the head and neck or the gastrointestinal tract, and those involving mediastinal structures
  b. Patients who have undergone radiation treatments to these areas
  c. Patients who are severely immunocompromised (e.g., AIDS, post-chemotherapy, steroid therapy)
  d. Patients who have progressive neuromuscular diseases (e.g., amyotrophic lateral sclerosis [ALS])
  e. Patients who have cerebrovascular disease (post-stroke)
  f. Patients who are experiencing medication-induced dystonic reactions
  g. Patients with respiratory compromise or who have recently been extubated
  h. Patients with a history of severe reflux, heartburn, or repeated pneumonia

Findings

- Excessive secretions, drooling
- Painful and/or uncoordinated swallowing
- Avoidance of food or beverages
- Choking, coughing, excessive throat-clearing during meals
- Increased respiratory rate or labored breathing during meals
- Increased congestion after meals
- Panting or other postures indicating difficulty in managing oral secretions and swallowing
- Whitish patches (plaques) in oral cavity (tongue, mucosal surface, gingiva) that scrape off and have a beefy red base
- Erythematous oral mucosa without plaques (atrophic candidiasis)
- Taste perversion

Evaluation

- History and systems review pertinent to upper gastrointestinal system, including sense of taste, quality and intensity of pain, difficulties with chewing and swallowing
- History of previous swallowing problems and dietary modifications
- History of changes in vocal pitch or new vocal breathiness (may indicate new vocal fold dysfunction)

- Examination of oropharynx: observe for signs of candida, other lesions, fit of dentures, odor (halitosis), posterior pharyngeal erythema indicating possible irritation from reflux, or pocketed food from an earlier meal
- Observe patient manage own secretions during history-taking, and observe patient during the act of swallowing
- Observe bedding for evidence of residue from previous meals on the pillow-case or sheets
- Review medications for possible dystonic reactions from phenothiazines, butyrophenones, etc. (e.g., prochlorperazine, chlorpromazine, haloperidol, droperidol)

Processes of Care

Practical

- Optimize positioning for drinking and eating (sitting if possible, or elevated head of bed)
- Frequent small sips or meals; crushed ice; refresh bedside beverages/ice frequently
- Alternate bites and sips to clear food from posterior pharynx
- Frequent rest breaks during meals
- Mouth care after each meal
- Have patient avoid excessively sour (acidic) or hot fluids/meals until symptoms remit. Soft, cool meals (yogurt, cottage cheese, pudding, ice cream) may be all that is tolerated
- Avoid mixed-consistency foods like stew as these take considerable coordination to chew and swallow the consistency mix (both solid and liquid components in a single bite)
- Speech Pathology consult to customize dietary consistency modifications, to develop compensatory postures/strategies to maximize eating safety, and to train caregivers
- Dietary/nutritionist consultation to maximize nutrition within parameters of the dysphagia

Biomedical

- For dystonia, if symptom-causing medication is still indicated, initiate therapy with diphenhydramine 25 to 50 mg PO/IV qid or benztropine 1 to 2 mg PO/IV qd or bid
- For painful oral candidiasis and mucositis, use opioid analgesics as needed to control pain until antifungal therapy has been effective; a 1:2:8 mixture of diphenhydramine elixir:lidocaine (2% to 4%): Maalox as a swish-and-swallow suspension provides temporary relief of symptoms and might lessen the need for opioid analgesics, especially prior to mealtimes
- Edema, inflammation, tumor burden: consider corticosteroids and H_2 blockers (potential benefit of corticosteroids must be balanced against associated risks of immunosuppression)

- For candidiasis, treat with:
  1. Topical treatment with clotrimazole 10-mg troches, 5 doses/day can be initiated, as symptoms and patient compliance allow
  2. If symptoms do not rapidly abate or patient compliance does not allow topical antifungal therapy, fluconazole 150 mg PO followed by 100 mg PO daily for 5 days
- Intractable oral bleeding: if available, apply topical thrombin to hemorrhagic areas; consider tranexamic acid 500 to 1,000 mg PO tid or aminocaproic acid 5 g PO followed by 1 g PO qid (see "Bleeding, Oozing, and Malodorous Lesions" earlier in this section)
- Severe halitosis should be treated to prevent reluctance to provide care, social isolation, humiliation, and nausea:
  1. Frequent prophylactic care (cleansing of dentures and oropharynx)
  2. Antimicrobial mouthwash or half-strength hydrogen peroxide gargle
  3. Metronidazole 250 to 500 mg PO tid or applied as a topical gel (0.75%), if feasible, to putrid necrotic or fungating lesions for control of anaerobic colonization (see "Bleeding, Oozing, and Malodorous Lesions" earlier in this section)
  4. Broad-spectrum antibiotics (e.g., trimethoprim-sulfa; cephalosporin) for foul-smelling, purulent bronchopulmonary sputum/secretions
  5. Treat reflux
  6. Elevate the head of the bed with low blocks if needed for reflux control

Goals/Outcomes

- Decrease pain
- Normalize swallowing and control of secretions as much as disease status allows
- Improve enjoyment of food and beverages
- Improve ability to talk
- Reduce social isolation, embarrassment, nausea

Documentation in the Medical Record

Initial Assessment

- History of difficulty with swallowing or managing secretions, choking
- Type and quantity of food/beverage intake causing both most problems and also best success
- Time of day problems exist (e.g., worse as the day progresses) if applicable
- Pain in mouth, throat, or mediastinum
- Physical examination findings
- Patient/caregiver ability to cope with symptoms/interventions
- Patient ability to ingest oral or buccal medications; possible need for liquid forms of pills/capsules and/or transdermal, SQ, or IV dosage forms

Interdisciplinary Progress Notes

- Interventions recommended, tried and outcomes
- Results of evaluations and caregiver observations

- Patient/caregiver difficulties with compliance
- Findings from repeat physical examinations

IDT Care Plan

- Specific interventions for each identified symptom
- Oral hygiene plan
- Contingency plans
- Planned modifications to any religious, spiritual, or other rituals needed because of the dysphagia/odynophagia
- Schedule of follow-up visits/examinations

Recommended Reading

Clarkson JE, Worthington HV, Furness S, McCabe M, Khalid T, Meyer S. Interventions for treating oral mucositis for patients with cancer receiving treatment. Cochrane Database Systematic Reviews. 2010;Aug 4(8):CD001973

Marik PE. Pulmonary aspiration syndromes. Current Opinion Pulmonary Medicine. 2011;17(3):148–154

Marlow C, Johnson J. A guide to managing the pain of treatment-related oral mucositis. Int J Palliat Nursing. 2005;11(7):338–345

Pollens R. Role of the speech language pathologist in palliative hospice care. J Palliat Med. 2004;7(5):694–702

Sciubba JJ. End of life considerations in the head and neck cancer patient. Oral Oncol. 2009;45:431–434

Edema: Peripheral Edema, Ascites, and Lymphedema

SITUATION: Peripheral edema, ascites, or lymphedema that results in physical or emotional distress or functional impairment or adds difficulty to caregiving

Causes

- Ascites and lymphedema
  - Primary neoplasm (ovary, breast, endometrium, colon, stomach, pancreas, bronchus, hepatobiliary)
  - Right heart failure
  - Metastasis to peritoneum or liver
  - Venous or lymphatic obstruction/occlusion due to neoplasm
  - Portal hypertension secondary to advanced liver disease
  - Chylous ascites (lymph plus emulsified fat and white blood cells) from lymphatic obstruction or abdominal lymphoma
  - Postsurgical or radiotherapy-induced lymphatic obstruction
- Peripheral edema
  - Hypoalbuminemia
  - Chronic steroid therapy
  - Renal failure

- Congestive heart failure
- Circulatory impairment from inadequate mobility/prolonged dependency
- Fluid overload from artificial nutrition
- Chronic peripheral vascular disease/post-thrombosis syndrome
- Cor pulmonale (right heart failure) due to advanced pulmonary disease
- Acute phlebitis
- Drug induced (e.g., NSAIDs, corticosteroids, cyclosporine)

Findings
- Ascites
  - Feelings of bloating, regurgitation, or reflux
  - Early satiety and nausea
  - Increased abdominal girth, shifting dullness, fluid wave, caput medusae (engorged venous plexus visible on abdominal wall in severe cases of portal hypertension)
  - Lower extremity/genital swelling
  - Orthopnea and dyspnea as ascites progresses
- Lymphedema or peripheral edema
  - Swelling of distal extremities with pitting of skin when gentle pressure is applied
  - Presence of fluid accumulation in dependent body parts (e.g., presacral area in bed-bound patients)
  - Unilateral extremity swelling in postsurgical or post-radiotherapy lymphedema
  - Tight and shiny skin with visible fluid extrusion in severe cases
  - Jugular venous distention
  - Pain with acute phlebitis
  - Electrolyte abnormalities

Evaluation
- Assess cardiovascular status (e.g., vital signs, cardiac rate, rhythm, murmurs, rubs, gallops, jugular veins, peripheral pulses, peripheral perfusion)
- Examine dependent body parts and extremities
- Auscultate lungs for rales, rubs, and decreased breath sounds
- Examine abdomen for findings of ascites
- Assess fluid balance (volume in, urine out), when appropriate; consider benefit versus burden of serum electrolyte and protein assessment
- Assess weight changes, when feasible
- Assess for tachypnea and respiratory distress
- Evaluate for symptoms of reflux
- Determine association between body position and physical signs and symptoms of distress

Processes of Care

Practical and Biomedical

- Ascites: Pharmacotherapy to reduce the ascitic burden should be tried, but effects may be marginal, especially in malignant ascites
    1. Diuretics
        a. Spironolactone 100 mg PO daily up to 200 mg bid. If needed, add:
        b. Furosemide 40 to 240 mg PO daily; continuous infusion of 100 mg/ 24 hr IV is an alternative; balance benefits against potential adverse effects, such as volume depletion and electrolyte disturbance
        c. Patients with soft edema who have failed to respond to medical management with diuretics can be treated with subcutaneous needle drainage
    2. Symptomatic ascites that is intractable to diuretic therapy and subcutaneous needle drainage may require large-volume paracentesis at the bedside, but relief is usually temporary
- If highly symptomatic ascites reaccumulates quickly and the patient is not imminently dying, discuss regarding the placement of a dialysis catheter for continuous drainage, acknowledging the burdens associated with such a procedure (transport to a day-surgery facility; discomfort from the operative procedure; risk of infection, occlusion, dislodgment)
- Peritoneo-venous shunting (PVS) may have a place in malignant ascites. The cytologic status of ascites should be considered in selection for PVS, as a shunt half-life is significantly greater in cytologically negative ascites; contraindications include loculated ascites, jaundice, infection, hemorrhagic ascites or ascitic fluid protein greater than 50 g/L, pseudomyxoma peritonei, and coagulopathy
- Lymphedema: Primary treatment consists of nonpharmacological approaches (e.g., postural support; maintaining range of motion with active or passive physical therapy, as tolerated; compression bandaging/gloves/stockings/pneumatic devices); diuretics (see "Air Hunger (Dyspnea)" earlier in this section) should be tried if symptoms are distressing, although responses to drug therapy are not generally very positive
- Peripheral edema
    - Review current diuretic and cardiac medications with physician, and adjust appropriately (see above)
    - Elevate legs prn unless contraindicated by compromised cardiac function
    - Turn and reposition recumbent patients q2hr as tolerated
    - Consider relative benefits/burdens of decreasing fluid intake
    - Consider need for daily potassium supplement when patient is on long-term diuretic therapy
    - Consider antibiotic therapy if cellulitis is present
    - Notify physician if findings of acute thrombophlebitis are present

Goals/Outcomes

- Reduce ascites, lymphedema, and peripheral edema to the greatest extent with the least invasive approaches possible in order to minimize physical and emotional distress, improve patient physical functioning, and facilitate caregiving

Documentation in the Medical Record

Initial Assessment

- Results of systems review and physical examination
- Intensity and types of physical and emotional distress, functional loss to patient imposed by ascites/lymphedema/peripheral edema
- Degree of burden imposed by untreated signs/symptoms on caregiver

Interdisciplinary Progress Notes

- Content of discussion regarding treatment options
- Types and results of interventions

IDT Care Plan

- Defined goals of therapies
- Specific interventions and contingency plans

Recommended Reading

Bar-Sela G, Omer A, Flechter E, et al. Treatment of lower extremity edema by subcutaneous drainage in palliative care of advanced cancer patients. Am J Hosp Palliat Care. 2010;27(4):272–275

Beng TS, Chin LE. Multiple subcutaneous puncture and stoma bag drainage for gross lower limb edema: A case report. J Palliat Med. 2010;13(8):1037–1038

Cheung DK, Raff JH. Selection of patients with malignant ascites for peritoneovenous shunting. Cancer 1982;50:1204–1209

Fischer DS. Abdominal paracentesis for malignant ascites. Arch Intern Med. 1979;139(2):235

Lam PT, Wong MS, Tse CY. Use of closed controlled subcutaneous drainage to manage chronic lower limb oedema in patients with advanced cancer. Hong Kong Med J. 2009;15(1):65–68

McCaffery J. Management of serous effusions. In: Lokick JJ, ed. Clinical Cancer Medicine. Boston, 1980, pp. 231–248

Straus AK, Roseman DL, Shapiro TM. Peritoneovenous shunting in the management of malignant ascites. Arch Surg 1979;114(4):489–491

Fatigue, Weakness (Aesthenia), and Excessive Sedation

SITUATION: The patient's quality of life is severely affected by fatigue, weakness, or diminished energy due to advancing disease

Causes

- Most chronic disease states in the far advanced stages (e.g., cancer, COPD, heart failure, renal failure, hepatic failure) lead to a state of aesthenia, characterized by chronic fatigue and weakness; these continue to be some of the most challenging symptoms to manage effectively, once pain is under control

- Catabolic nutritional state due to disease factors
- Hypoxemia or inadequate oxygen-carrying capacity (decreased red cell mass)
- Clinical depression should be ruled out since the symptoms of depression may mimic aesthenia (see "Depression" earlier in this section)
- Medications: Anticholinergics, antihistamines, benzodiazepines and other sleep aids, neuroleptics commonly cause fatigue and sedation; antihypertensive therapy that may have been appropriate previously may cause excessive reduction in blood pressure in debilitated patients with weight loss, resulting in marked fatigue and postural hypotension
- Excessive use of alcohol may go unrecognized, especially in the elderly, or may be viewed as benign in chronically ill patients
- Boredom: Absence of stimulation is very common in homebound and especially bedridden patients, and can mimic depression

Findings

- Weakness, lethargy, fatigue, hypersomnolence after minimal or no activity

Evaluation

Biomedical

- Simple measures should be used to find and treat reversible or easily treatable causes of severe fatigue, lethargy, and weakness (e.g., metabolic disturbances, anemia, hypoxemia) when the context is appropriate (i.e., life expectancy will allow meaningful benefit from testing and therapeutic intervention); in patients with rapid decline from life-limiting diseases, the luxury of an exhaustive evaluation is not always feasible or in the patient's best interest; in these cases, or where reversible processes are not present or specifically directed therapies are not possible, empiric therapy is indicated
- Review current medications and determine if there are any changes that, on balance, might lead to overall benefits
- Evaluate muscle tone and strength; unless myopathic weakness is the result of ongoing corticosteroid therapy, this class of drugs can palliate symptoms of weakness and fatigue for a short time (days to weeks)

Psychosocial/Spiritual

- Determine patient/caregiver perceptions and level of distress imposed by degree of fatigue and weakness
- Determine to what degree important short-term goals are being impeded by symptoms

Processes of Care

Biomedical

- Consider and discuss benefits and burdens of red cell transfusion if anemia is a likely contributing cause of symptoms
- Use supplemental oxygen only if a therapeutic trial proves beneficial when hypoxemia is determined to be the cause of symptoms

- In patients with heart failure, review medical management and determine if there are any adjustments in cardiotropic drugs that may improve end-organ perfusion, balancing benefits/burdens and patient preferences
- Palliative pharmacotherapy using psychostimulants can be tried; the use of dextroamphetamine or methylphenidate may be especially useful in balancing therapeutic analgesic effects of opioids against excessive daytime sedation; modafinil has also been reported to be beneficial, although its cost is appreciably higher than that of other psychostimulants; it should be considered if other modalities are not well tolerated; close follow-up and monitoring for incipient signs of psychosis, agitation, or sleep disturbance are obligatory when instituting these drug therapies:
  1. Dextroamphetamine 2.5 mg PO every morning to start, or
  2. Methylphenidate 2.5 mg PO every morning to start, or

NOTE: These medications can be titrated upward as needed and can be used as often as three or four times per day, depending on each patient's needs and response to therapy. There is some evidence that small doses throughout the day may be more effective than morning and midday dosing and do not lead to insomnia as has been traditionally thought.

  3. Modafinil 200 mg PO every morning

Psychosocial/Spiritual

- Provide realistic information about the natural history of the disease process being experienced, with aesthenia being a usual and expected consequence
- Help organize the patient/caregiver routines to conserve energy and pace activities. Address the potential value of hiring aides
- Review the role of energy-sparing devices such as a walker, wheelchair, or motorized scooter; patients may be reluctant to use such devices because they visibly represent loss of functional capacity, so this may be an ongoing discussion and reorientation of values in order to preserve dignity
- Help set limits on social visits if they seem to be more exhausting than helpful
- Help reset goals to a level that is more attainable based on the patient's capabilities
- Consider occupational therapy evaluation to determine if there is any form of stimulation that might be beneficial; use volunteers to carry on such a program to counteract boredom
- Formal rehabilitation programs may improve function in patients with cancer and cardiopulmonary disease and may be appropriate for patients with a more extended prognosis

Goals/Outcomes

- Maximize patient energy based on the course of disease, in keeping with patient preferences
- Decreased frustration with clinical circumstances beyond patient/caregiver/professional control

- Patient feels free from having to perform at an unrealistic level of expectation
- Identify short-term goals (whatever they are—even simply "being") that are attainable and lead the patient to feel that his/her existence has value

Documentation in the Medical Record

Initial Assessment

- Description of patient's level of fatigue, functional capabilities
- Determination if goals and expectations are realistic
- Degree of acceptance versus frustration with clinical circumstances
- Identification of factors contributing to fatigue, weakness (pacing, length of social visits, structure and schedule of activities throughout the day)

Interdisciplinary Progress Notes

- Content of discussions, ongoing evaluations, interventions
- Results of interventions

IDT Care Plan

- Specific interventions and role of IDT members in helping to manage coping issues

Recommended Reading

Escalante CP, Manzullo EF. Cancer-related fatigue: The approach and treatment. J Gen Intern Med. 2009;24(Suppl 2):412–416

Hardy SE. Methylphenidate for treatment of depressive symptoms, apathy, and fatigue in medically ill older adults and terminally ill adults. Am J Geriatr Pharmacother. 2009;7(1):34–59

Minton O, Richardson A, Sharpe M, Hotopf M, Stone P. Drug therapy for the management of cancer-related fatigue. Cochrane Database of Systematic Reviews. 2010; 7. Art. No.: CD006704

Rabkin JG, McElhiney MC, Rabkin R, McGrath P. Modafinil treatment for fatigue in patients with HIV/AIDS: A placebo controlled study. J Clin Psychiatry. 2010;71(6):707–715

Yennurajalingam S, Palmer JL, Chacko R, Bruera E. Factors associated with response to methylphenidate in advances cancer patients. Oncologist. 2011;16: 246–253

Fever and Diaphoresis

SITUATION: Fever and/or diaphoresis associated with terminal illness

Causes

- Infection
- Tumor-related pyrexia (i.e., from release of pro-inflammatory cytokines such as TNF alpha; interleukins [IL-1, IL-6])

- Tumor-related (paraneoplastic) nocturnal afebrile diaphoresis (night sweats); often associated with anorexia-cachexia as a symptom cluster (syndrome)
  - Lymphoma
  - Certain lung cancers
- Drug-induced afebrile diaphoresis (e.g., morphine)
- Central nervous system metastasis or primary neoplasm
- Drug- or transfusion-related pyrogenic reaction
- Dehydration
- Graft-versus-host disease (GVHD)

Findings

- Elevated body temperature (above 100.5° F orally, 99.5° F axillary, 101.5° F rectally)
- Flushed warm skin, generalized aching, irritability
- Tachycardia
- Altered mental status (decreased level of consciousness or agitation/restlessness, fitful sleep)
- Diaphoresis (sweating) with or without fever

Evaluation

- Systems review and physical examination to rule out infection (e.g., urinary tract, respiratory tract, cellulitis)
- Stage and extent of disease in relation to cause of fever/diaphoresis
- Recent medication change as potential cause of fever/diaphoresis

Processes of Care

Practical

- Increase room air circulation and give cool sponge baths
- Cool wet towels or ice packs to groin and axilla for temperature above 103° F as symptoms dictate and if tolerated
- Remove heavy bed clothes and bedding
- Provide mouth care: use toothette dipped in fluid of choice to moisten mouth and apply lip balm to keep lips from cracking

Biomedical

- Empiric broad-spectrum antibiotic therapy ONLY if occult or obvious infection is suspected AND symptoms are a cause of significant discomfort or a major burden to caregivers (e.g., necessity for frequent bedding changes)
- Pharmacotherapeutic approaches

  1. Antipyretics
     a. Acetaminophen 5 to 10 mg/kg PO/PR q4–6hr around the clock, or
     b. NSAIDs (e.g., ibuprofen 10 mg/kg PO q8hr or naproxen sodium 4 mg/kg PO q8hr)

2. Treatment of rigors (shaking chills) is empiric. Some recommended approaches are:
   a. Meperidine 0.25 to 0.5 mg/kg IV/IM/SQ prn *(NOTE: this is an exception to the usual injunction against the use of meperidine)*, or
   b. Promethazine 12.5 to 25 mg PO/IM/IV or 25 to 50 mg PR q6–8hr prn
3. For suspected metastasis-induced diaphoresis (e.g., liver metastasis) or morphine-induced sweating:
   a. Dexamethasone 2 mg PO, or
   b. Indomethacin 50 mg PR q12hr
   c. Cannabinoids (e.g., nabilone 1 mg PO qd or bid)
4. For prevention of macerated skin:
   a. Zinc oxide paste applied to intertriginous areas and other at-risk sites

Goals/Outcomes

- Reduce fever- and diaphoresis-associated discomfort and distress
- Decrease sleep disruption
- Minimize caregiving burden

Documentation in the Medical Record

Initial Assessment

- Body temperature and associated signs and symptoms of fever
- Timing of fever, diaphoresis (day/night)
- Interventions (and results) attempted by caregiver
- Differential diagnosis based on history and physical examination

Interdisciplinary Progress Notes

- Effect of interventions on symptoms

IDT Care Plan

- Specific interventions and contingency plans

Recommended Reading

Maida V. Nabilone for the treatment of paraneoplastic night sweats: A report of four cases. J Palliat Med. 2008;11(6):929–934

Meremikwu MM, Oyo-Ita A. Physical methods versus drug placebo or no treatment for managing fever in children. Cochrane Database of Systematic Reviews. 2003; 2. Art. No.: CD004264

Hiccups

SITUATION: Pain or discomfort and exhaustion due to persistent hiccups

Causes

- Gastric dysmotility with distention due to extrinsic obstruction or intrinsic disease

- Phrenic or vagus nerve irritation due to tumor or inflammation
- Arrhythmia-induced syncope has been reported as both the cause and the effect of hiccups
- Congenital malformations, malignancies, multiple sclerosis
- Cerebral neoplasms, metastasis or other central nervous system disorders (e.g., cerebrovascular disease)
- Recurrent laryngeal nerve irritation (mass lesions in neck, goiter, laryngitis)
- Metabolic disturbances (e.g., uremia, hypocalcemia, hyponatremia, fever, hypocarbia, hyperglycemia, hypokalemia)
- Sepsis
- Reflux esophagitis
- Manifestation of anxiety disorder

Findings

- Disruption of social interactions, eating, sleeping
- "Heartburn" or other chest pain (from reflux or muscle strain)
- Aspiration-induced chronic cough, pneumonitis
- Anxiety, aerophagia

Evaluation

Biomedical

- Systems review and physical examination for disease-related etiology as described earlier
- Metabolic evaluation in patients with an extended life expectancy where specific interventions to remediate the disorder are feasible should be discussed with the physician, IDT, and patient
- Effect of hiccups on pain, sleep, significant fatigue or depression
- Association of hiccups to secondary disorders such as reflux and aspiration
- Determine relationship of hiccups episodes to position, medication use, and type of food intake

Psychosocial

- Assess anxiety and "air swallowing" (aerophagia) as well as relationship of hiccups to sleep; hiccups that occur ONLY during wakefulness point to psychological causes

Process of Care Delivery

Practical

- Nonpharmacological management techniques often suffice, but they may require repetition; these include various means of trying to stimulate nasopharyngeal reflexes and associated cranial nerves involved in the hiccup reflex arc; for instance:
  - Forcible traction on the tongue
  - Swallowing or applying granulated sugar under the tongue
  - Gargling with water, sipping ice water, biting on a lemon

- Insertion of a small flexible catheter gently through the nose into the posterior pharynx
- Elevating the uvula with a cotton-tipped applicator
- Drinking from the far side of a glass (difficult for very ill patients to understand or carry out)
- Cold application to the back of the neck
- Breathing into paper bag
- Elevate the head of the bed, or support patient in a semirecumbent position with pillows/bolsters, especially after meals
- Experiment with position changes to determine if any one position offers relief (e.g., lateral)
- Acupuncture (including near-infrared irradiation of acupoints)

Biomedical

- Adjunctive use of pharmacotherapy to maintain a "remission" from recurrent bouts of hiccups might be necessary; all of the following drug regimens have been found to be effective, but each patient requires a trial-and-error approach; start with the therapy that is least toxic and least likely to induce side effects (this also depends on each patient's unique set of circumstances) and then try the next treatment on the list if needed:.
  1. Chlorpromazine 25 to 50 mg IV (only FDA-approved medication for hiccups; effective in 80% of cases)
  2. Metoclopramide 10 to 20 mg PO/IV q8hr if there is delayed gastric emptying *without bowel obstruction*
  3. Simethicone and/or charcoal-containing antacids prn
  4. Haloperidol 1 to 5 mg PO/IV qid, or chlorpromazine 10 to 25 mg PO or 25-mg suppository PR qid
  5. Prednisone 1 mg/kg/day, then taper, if hepatomegaly or tumor effect is suspected as etiology
  6. Phenytoin 100 mg PO bid
  7. Valproic acid and carbamazepine have been effective when used in typical anticonvulsant doses
  8. Gabapentin has been shown to be effective where CNS lesions are present and in some other etiologic groups, including in cancer patients
  9. Baclofen, a centrally acting muscle relaxant, administered at 10 mg PO up to four times a day; particularly useful in patients for whom other agents are contraindicated (e.g., those with renal impairment)
  10. Other drugs that have been successful based on case reports include edrophonium, dexamethasone, amantadine, and nifedipine

Psychosocial

- Treat anxiety as described in "Agitation and Anxiety" earlier in this section

Goals/Outcomes

- Reduce or eliminate episodes of hiccupping to the extent possible without incurring additional symptom burdens from treatment
- Provide periods of uninterrupted rest and sleep

- Improve social interaction and ability to partake of meals as per patient preference
- Eliminate "heartburn" and risk of aspiration

Documentation in the Medical Record

Initial Assessment

- Frequency and duration of hiccup episodes with inciting and relieving factors, if identified
- Putative etiology of hiccups, if identified
- Effect of hiccups on social interaction, meals, pain, sleep, mood

Interdisciplinary Progress Notes

- Effects of interventions

IDT Care Plan

- Decisions regarding value of further medical workup
- Specific interventions (nonmedical and medical) with contingency and follow-up plans

Recommended Reading

Chang CC, Chang YC, Chang ST, et al. Efficacy of near-infrared irradiation on intractable hiccup in custom-set acupoints: evidence-based analysis of treatment outcome and associated factors. Scand J Gastroenterol. 2008;43(5):538–544

Marinella MA. Diagnosis and management of hiccups in the patient with advanced cancer. J Support Oncol. 2009;7(4):122–127

Ong AM, Tan CS, Foo MW, Kee TY. Gabapentin for intractable hiccups in a patient undergoing peritoneal dialysis. Perit Dial Int. 2008;28(6):667–668

Suh WM, Krishnan SC. Violent hiccups: an infrequent cause of bradyarrhythmias. West J Emerg Med. 2009;10(3):176–177

Turkyilmaz A, Eroglu A. Use of baclofen in the treatment of esophageal stent-related hiccups. Ann Thorac Surg. 2008;85(1):328–330

Wilcox SK, Garry A, Johnson MJ. Novel use of amantadine: to treat hiccups. J Pain Symptom Manage. 2009;38(3):460–465

Imminent Death

SITUATION: Rapid decline in medical condition with associated signs and symptoms of imminent death

Findings

- Overall deterioration of bodily functions/homeostasis with accompanying general systems failure—all systems weaken
- Cardiac/progressive circulatory failure
  - Tachycardia that may degenerate to bradyarrhythmias
  - Hypotension
  - Weak peripheral pulses
  - Cool, mottled extremities

- Renal insufficiency
  - Decreased urinary output
- Pulmonary failure
  - Tachypnea with periods of apnea (Cheyne-Stokes respirations)
  - Increased use of accessory muscles for respiration
  - Terminal congestion ("death rattle")
- Deterioration of cognition and higher brain functions/mental status changes
  - Progressive lethargy (obtundation)
  - Social withdrawal
  - Speaking to being(s) unseen by others in attendance
  - Picking at bedclothes or in the air
  - Agitation or restlessness

Evaluation

- Assess the need for support by various members of the IDT, depending on areas of expertise, especially the need for spiritual and bereavement support
- Anticipate the mode of death in order to prepare family/caregiver
- Assess for behaviors suggestive of pain, dyspnea, fear
- Determine whether bladder emptying is taking place
  - Literature supports non-invasive bladder ultrasound as a new standard of care
- Determine type of secretions causing "death rattle"
  - Oral: clear, relatively thin, not particularly malodorous
  - Bronchial: purulent, relatively thick, fetid odor
- Assess caregiver's level of comfort, capability, and competency with basic care (e.g., hygiene, positioning, suctioning, medication administration)
- Determine if post-death plans have been made (funeral home, etc.)
- Review with caregiver whether important family members/significant others need to be or want to be notified of patient status
- Determine whether current level of care is sufficient to manage patient symptoms and/or support caregiver

Processes of Care

Practical and Biomedical

- Review and ensure provision of basic processes of physical care: oropharyngeal care (lips, teeth, oral mucosa), bathing, positioning, skin care, suctioning, medication administration
- Ensure adequacy of urinary drainage, if urine is still being produced
- Nonpurulent secretions: a patient's inability to control or swallow secretions can be managed by positioning and having suction available for use by the caregivers, coupled with the use of drying agents when more bronchial or respiratory sounds are disturbing to those close to the patient; there are many choices for palliative pharmacotherapy; convenience, cost, and potential for undesirable (adverse or toxic) effects should lead to the most rational

first choice, with appropriate monitoring and adjustments made based on response. A recent study showed that any of the therapies below can be equally effective compared to placebo.

1. Transdermal scopolamine patches: each patch delivers 1 mg of scopolamine per 24 hours for 3 days; more than one patch may be required, titrating therapeutic effects against potential side effects, which include sedation and delirium (tertiary amine, does cross blood–brain barrier and may cause CNS adverse side effects)

2. Hyoscyamine 0.125 mg SL q1–2hr prn (tertiary amine, does cross blood–brain barrier and may cause CNS adverse side effects)

3. Scopolamine 0.3 to 0.6 mg SQ prn (tertiary amine, does cross blood–brain barrier and may cause CNS adverse side effects)

4. Glycopyrrolate 0.2 mg IV/SQ prn (quaternary ammonium, does not cross blood–brain barrier)

5. Atropine 1 to 2mg /SQ/SL/nebulized q4hr or prn

- Purulent secretions should also be managed with positioning and suctioning, but drying agents may not be particularly helpful; a single IV injection (if IV access is available) of a broad-spectrum antibiotic (e.g., a cephalosporin such as cefotaxime 500 to 1,000 mg /IV) has been shown to sufficiently decrease the bacterial count with accompanying elimination of malodorous character of bronchial secretions; this effect may last for days, allowing a much-reduced caregiving burden and eliminating a barrier to physical closeness; furthermore, if pneumonia is thought to be present, then a full course of antibiotics may actually increase comfort

- Restlessness or agitation: refer to "Agitation and Anxiety" earlier in this section

- Change route of medication administration if oral route has been in effect and this route is no longer feasible: consult with physician/pharmacist as necessary for dosage conversions/formulations

- Notify the primary care physician, as well as appropriate consulting physicians and/or hospice physician of status, depending on expressed preferences

- Institute appropriate level of care to ensure adequate symptom management and essential care

Psychosocial/Spiritual/Practical

- Continue to reassure patient through verbal communication and touch, even if there is no direct evidence of understanding or acknowledgment by the patient

- Offer emotional support to caregiver, answer questions, and provide situation-specific information about processes of dying, including:
  - Possible occurrence of death during turning or other basic care
  - Possible occurrence of death during transport to another care facility if that becomes the choice/preference/necessity
  - Possible occurrence of a postmortem audible exhalation

- Help to distinguish and give reassurance to the caregiver and others in attendance about the difference between pain/suffering and terminal vocalizations, if present

- Reassure caregiver/family that discontinuation of food/fluids when patient is no longer interested or responsive is "best care," reducing the burden to patient
- Institute appropriate level of care to ensure adequate patient and caregiver support
- Help to notify designated family, friends, clergy, etc., per patient/caregiver preferences
- Review contingency plans for caregiver coping/support (e.g., 24-hour hospice telephone number in order to prevent a "panic" reaction such as dialing 911)
- Review information on procedure to follow after death, including disposition of body to funeral home or other prearrangements
- Provide mouth and eye care: use toothette dipped in fluid of choice to moisten mouth and apply lip balm to keep lips from cracking; use artificial tears to moisten eyes, if open, and warm water and soft cloth to clear mucus/crusting
- Facilitate and respect rituals as specified by patient/family

Goals/Outcomes

- The dying process and death itself will occur with maximal comfort and with dignity
- Caregiver/family will experience a sense of enduring emotional comfort from the experience of their loved one dying in a nurturing/caring environment and in a manner that respected their preferences to the greatest extent possible

Documentation in the Medical Record

Initial Assessment
- Determination that on initial assessment the patient is imminently dying
- Focus of the evaluation should be on biomedical/psychosocial/practical/spiritual findings and preparation for death

Interdisciplinary Progress Notes
- Ongoing and progressive physical signs and symptoms
- Coping by caregiver/family
- Description of instructions, preparations, interventions
- Results of interventions

IDT Care Plan
- Specific interventions planned
- Contingency plans and schedule of follow-up by various members of IDT
- Updated bereavement plan

Recommended Reading

Currow DC, Abernethy AP, eds. Respiratory problems. In: Current Opinion in Supportive & Palliative Care. 2009;3(2):120–124

Martin JL, et al. Systematic review and meta-analysis of methods of diagnostic assessment for urinary incontinence. Neurourology and Urodynamics. 2006; 25:674–684

Newman DK, Gaines T, Snare E. Innovation in bladder assessment: use of technology in extended care. J Gerontological Nursing. 2005;31(12):33–41

Muir JC, von Gunten CF. Antisecretory agents in gastrointestinal obstruction. Clin Geriatr Med. 2000;16(2):327–334

van der Steen JT, Ooms ME, van der Wal G, Ribbe MW. Pneumonia: the demented patient's best friend? Discomfort after starting or withholding antibiotic treatment. J Am Geriatr Soc. 2002;50:1681–1688

Wildiers H, Demeulenaere P, Clement P, Menten J. Treatment of death rattle in dying patients. Belgian J Med Oncol. 2008;2:275–279

Insomnia and Nocturnal Restlessness

SITUATION: Disturbed sleep or significant alteration in sleep pattern interfering with patient sense of well-being or adding to caregiver burden

Sleep disorders are common in the general population and many studies indicate they are even more frequent in hospice and palliative care patients. Sleep disorders may be described by patients as delayed onset of sleep (increased sleep latency), difficulty maintaining sleep, early awakening, or a combination of these disturbances.

Although sleep problems are common in the hospice and palliative care patient population, they may be under-reported and under-recognized in these patients for a variety of reasons. Patients may believe sleep problems are inevitable or unavoidable concomitants of serious illness, or believe that their sleep symptoms are inconsequential compared to the severity of their chronic, progressive disease. In addition, patients with cognitive or communication impairments may not be able to report their sleep symptoms. Poor sleep has a great impact on mood, coping abilities, pain tolerance, interpersonal relations, appetite, energy, and overall sense of well-being. It is therefore important to regularly inquire of patients and caregivers whether patients are experiencing problems with sleep.

Causes

- Physical symptoms and dysfunctions may contribute to sleep disturbances:
  - Pain
  - Urinary retention
  - Constipation
  - Dyspnea
  - Heartburn
  - Nausea
  - Pruritus
  - Diarrhea
  - Urinary frequency
  - Abdominal distention from ascites or tumor burden
- A preexisting sleep disorder may continue to cause symptoms and may be worsened by the illness or therapy; obstructive and central sleep apnea may be worsened by prescribed opioids, anticholinergics, or benzodiazepines

- Emotional, psychological, or spiritual concerns may cause nighttime rumination and worry and may impair sleep
- CNS-stimulating medications may disturb sleep (decongestants, methylxanthines, selective serotonin reuptake inhibitors, psychostimulants, corticosteroids); opioids prescribed for pain may cause daytime somnolence and thereby interfere with nighttime sleep
- Chemotherapy and radiation therapy are associated with daytime fatigue and disrupted nighttime sleep patterns
- Use of illicit drugs, alcohol, or tobacco or withdrawal from these substances may disrupt normal sleep patterns
- Environmental factors in the living area may impair sound sleep (e.g., noisy equipment such as oxygen concentrators; nighttime caregiving needs that awaken the patient; an uncomfortable bed; intrusive catheters, SQ or IV lines)
- Inadequate sleep hygiene: Good sleep hygiene practices normally include reserving the bedroom and bed for intimate activities and sleep only; as patients become weaker, however, they may spend the majority of the day and perform their daily activities (reading, watching television, listening to music) in the bedroom and in bed; they can no longer adhere to this component of good sleep hygiene
- Recent hospitalization: In the hospital, patients' sleep is often interrupted by patient care activities and bright lights during the night; this disturbs the normal sleep–wake cycle; when patients return home, they often have trouble reestablishing their previous sleep patterns

Findings

- Complaint of poor sleep, exhaustion (by patient and/or caregiver(s), family members)
- Cognitively functional and expressive patients may be able to report on sleep history, but many patients are not aware of the details of sleep disturbance or nocturnal behaviors, requiring reliance on caregiver reports and/or daytime symptoms
- Moodiness, grouchiness, emotional lability/volatility
- Daytime sedation, nighttime restlessness
- Caregiver fatigue, frustration, exasperation, depression

Evaluation

Biomedical

- Sleep history
  - Onset of sleep, frequency of wakening, total duration, daytime sleep; use sleep assessment questionnaires and sleep diaries, if appropriate
    — Pittsburgh Sleep Quality Index (http://www.sleep.pitt.edu/content. asp?id=1484&subid=2316)
    — Sleep diaries
    — (http://science-education.nih.gov/supplements/nih3/sleep/guide/nih_ sleep_masters.pdf)

— National Sleep Foundation sleep diary (http://sleep.buffalo.edu/sleep-diary.pdf)
— Epworth Sleepiness Scale (http://www.stanford.edu/~dement/epworth.html)

- Assess for inadequately treated symptoms of primary and related disease processes, especially pain and dyspnea (orthopnea)
- Evaluate for signs or symptoms of primary sleep disorder (restless legs syndrome, other movement disorder, obstructive sleep apnea, night terrors)
- Review prescribed medications and treatments and evaluate their effect on sleep.
- Review use of alcohol, tobacco, non-prescribed medications, and illicit medications and substances whose use may have increased or decreased
- Explore how the sleep disorder is affecting the patient and caregivers' function

Psychosocial/Spiritual

- Explore emotional, psychological, social, and spiritual concerns and distress that may impair sleep
- Get corroboration of sleep pattern from others in home (especially if patient has impaired cognition or communication)
- Determine patient and caregivers' expectations of acceptable sleep pattern
- Assess caregiver fatigue and coping strategies

Practical

- Assess sleeping area and environmental factors (bed and bedding/pillows, noise, temperature, privacy)
- Assess safety if patient is up at night (night light, proximity of commode, obstacles, etc.)

Processes of Care

Practical/Psychosocial/Spiritual

- Progressive relaxation techniques/exercises as appropriate (http://www.umm.edu/sleep/relax_tech.htm#a)
- Small carbohydrate bedtime snack/beverage (e.g., warm milk with favorite flavoring)
- Presleep talk, storytelling, music
- Ensure a safe environment.
- Maximize daytime activities and stimulation (use of volunteers, etc.):
  - Components of sleep hygiene (some of these measures may not be applicable to a debilitated, bed-bound patient):
    — Maintain a regular sleep routine
    — Avoid naps if possible
    — Do not stay in bed awake for more than 5 to 10 minutes
    — Do not drink caffeine late in the day
    — Do not watch television in bed or read in bed
    — Avoid substances that interfere with sleep
    — Exercise regularly (if possible)

— Have a quiet, comfortable bedroom
— If patient is a "clock watcher" at night, hide the clock
— Have a comfortable pre-bedtime routine
— Consider sleep restriction; for patients who are not bed-bound, encourage them to stay in bed for only the number of hours that they are able to sleep; if unable to sleep they should get out of bed and engage in a quiet relaxing activity until sleepy again; patient should retire to bed 15 minutes earlier every night until the preferred sleep duration is achieved
- Increase level of care if caregiver exhaustion or inadequate coping
- Supportive counseling for mood disturbance (anxiety, depression)
  - Facilitate expression of fears, worries, "unfinished business"

Biomedical

- Optimize medical management of contributing causes of pain, dyspnea, hypoxia, urinary frequency, GERD, etc.
- Evaluate and treat or mitigate primary sleep disorders (obstructive sleep apnea, restless legs syndrome):
  - Symptomatic management of restless legs
    — Low-dose sedating tricyclic antidepressants (e.g., amitriptyline 10 mg PO HS)
    — Low-dose Sinemet (carbidopa/levodopa; initial dose 10 mg PO HS)
    — Gabapentin (initial dose 100 mg PO HS)
    — Ropinirole (initial dose 0.25 mg PO HS)
- Adjust medication schedule to the extent feasible to eliminate daytime sedation and nocturnal stimulation
- Treat anxiety, depression if not responsive to nonpharmacological interventions
- Advise and educate patient about hazards of illicit substance use, alcohol and tobacco use, or recent reduction in use, and over-the-counter medication use
- Pharmacotherapy

NOTE: There is a risk of increasing confusion, obtundation, daytime sedation, balance disturbances, etc., with the addition of any CNS depressant, especially in the frail elderly; close monitoring and low-dose titration are important.

- Benzodiazepines: These medications decrease the time to sleep onset and prolong the first and second stages of sleep; short- or medium-acting agents are preferred because they minimize daytime sleepiness and are less likely to cause complex sleep-related behaviors; most benzodiazepines interact with inhibitors of CYP3A4 such as macrolide antibiotics; concurrent administration with CYP3A4 inhibitors or with alcohol or other CNS depressants, including certain opioids (e.g., fentanyl) may increase the CNS depressant effects of benzodiazepines
  - Short-acting agents
    — Triazolam 0.125 to 0.25 mg
    — Oxazepam 10 to 30 mg

- Intermediate-acting agents
  - Estazolam 1 to 2 mg
  - Lorazepam 1 to 5 mg
  - Temazepam 15 to 30 mg
- Benzodiazepine receptor agonists
  - Zaleplon (ultrashort-acting) 5 to 20 mg
  - Zolpidem (short-acting) 5 to 10 mg
  - Eszopiclone (intermediate duration) 1 to 3 mg
- Melatonin receptor agonists
  - Ramelteon (short-acting) 8 mg (avoid administration with a high-fat meal)
- Sedating antidepressants
  - These agents can be used for sleep due to significant sedating effects; anti-cholinergic effects must be carefully monitored
    - Amitriptyline 10 to 25 mg PO HS; titrate as needed
    - Doxepin 10 to 25 mg PO HS; titrate as needed
    - Trazodone 25 to 50 mg PO HS; titrate as needed
    - Mirtazapine 15 to 45 mg
- Antihistamines
  - This class of agents is best avoided due to anticholinergic side effects such as dry mouth and urinary retention; in addition they may cause mental clouding and ataxia, particularly in elderly patients
- Alcohol
  - Patients may use alcohol to induce sleep, but this should be discouraged because alcohol initially induces CNS depression and sleep, but it can cause rebound excitation and insomnia; in addition, alcohol may provoke gastroesophageal reflux and may have a diuretic effect, both of which can disrupt sleep
- Natural and herbal remedies
  - There are no clearly proven remedies in this category; the purity and optimum dose of these remedies have not been established
- Nocturnal delirium ("sundowning")
  - If nocturnal delirium is suspected, precipitating factors should be promptly sought and treated
  - Consider the possibility that alcohol or drug withdrawal may be producing the symptoms; patients may need treatment for withdrawal syndrome
  - While reversible medical causes are being assessed and treated, behavioral interventions should begin:
    - Patients should have a predictable routine
    - Extraneous stimuli should be minimized
    - Lighting should be improved to reduce confusion and allow patients who may have impaired sight to see familiar surroundings
    - Ensure safety of the environment
    - Ensure (when patient's physical status permits) adequate food and fluid

- — Assess for presence of urinary retention or constipation
- — Provide for dry clothing and adequate warmth or coolness
- — Constantly reassure and reorient
- For nocturnal delirium/agitation not responsive to nonpharmacological treatments, low doses of sedating,antipsychotic agents may be helpful:
  - Chlorpromazine 25 mg PO HS
  - Haloperidol 0.5 to 2 mg PO HS
  - Risperidone 0.25 to 2 mg PO qd

Goals/Outcomes

- Normalize patient sleep patterns
- Relieve distressing nocturnal symptoms
- Relieve caregiver burden during nocturnal hours

Documentation in the Medical Record

Initial Assessment

- Sleep patterns and symptoms of disturbed sleep
- Evaluation of causative factors
- Medication review
- Impact of sleep disturbance on patient and caregiver
- Interventions
- Effectiveness of interventions

Interdisciplinary Progress Notes

- Ongoing identification of contributing factors
- Results of interventions and adjustment of care plan

IDT Care Plan

- Nonpharmacological and pharmacological interventions
- Psychological, social, spiritual supports offered
- Prevention of caregiver "burnout"
- Plans for patient safety

Recommended Reading

Cohen-Mansfield J, Garfinkel D, Lipsona S. Melatonin for the treatment of sundowning in elderly persons with dementia—a preliminary study. Arch Gerontol Geriatrics. 2000;31(1):65–76

Mercadante S, Girelli D, Casuccio. Sleep disorders in advanced cancer patients: Prevalence and factors associated. Supportive Care in Cancer. 2004;12(5):355–359

Morin CM. Measuring outcomes in randomized clinical trials of insomnia treatments. Sleep Medicine Reviews. 2003;7(3):263–279

Ohayon MM. Epidemiology of insomnia: What we know and what we still need to learn. Sleep Medicine Reviews. 2002;6(2):97–111

Staedt J, Stoppe G. Treatment of rest-activity disorders in dementia and special focus on sundowning. Int J Geriatric Psychiatry. 2005;20(6):507–511

Volicer L, Harper D, Manning B, Goldstein R, Satlin A. Sundowning and circadian rhythms in Alzheimer's disease. Am J Psychiatry. 2001;158:704–711

Nausea and Vomiting

SITUATION: Recurrent or chronic nausea and/or vomiting

The physiology of nausea and vomiting involves multiple areas, neurotransmitters, pathways, and targets within the CNS and periphery that ultimately trigger activity in the vomiting center of the brain. These include the chemoreceptor trigger zone (CTZ), which involves dopamine, serotonin, and neurokinin; the cortex, which involves acetylcholine, serotonin, and histamine; peripheral pathways, which involve serotonin, norepinephrine, and acetylcholine; and vestibular activation, which involves acetylcholine and histamine. The complexity of this "system" allows for activation by a wide variety of mechanical and chemical stimuli, but conversely it also allows therapeutic intercession by a wide variety of agents.

Causes

Biomedical

- Visceral or gastrointestinal tract disorders (e.g., malignancy, bowel obstruction, ileus, constipation)
- CNS disturbances (e.g., neoplasm, increased intracranial pressure)
- Chemical triggers (e.g., odors, tastes, drugs)
- Vestibular disturbances
- Metabolic disturbances (e.g., hypercalcemia, hyperglycemia, uremia, infection)
- Mechanical triggers (e.g., gagging from coughing, hiccuping, retained secretions)

Psychosocial

- Conditioned response to situational/environmental/emotional/sensory stimuli
- Anxiety related to anticipation of nausea and/or vomiting

Findings

Biomedical

- Continuous or episodic nausea with or without vomiting
- Passive or projectile vomiting independent of or associated with food/fluid or medication intake

Psychosocial

- Varying degrees of withdrawal, fatigue, depressed mood, anxiety, aversion to triggering factors
- Varying degrees of acceptance, frustration, aversion by caregiver

Evaluation

Biomedical

- Systems review and physical examination to assess for:
  - Distention, bloating, evidence of bowel obstruction, peptic ulcer/gastritis/esophagitis, severe constipation or impaction

- Hepatomegaly
- Evidence of elevated intracranial pressure (papilledema, headache, altered mental status, spontaneous projectile vomiting)
- Dehydration
- Oropharyngeal examination (dentures, thrush, hyperreactive gag reflex)
- Medication review with attention to emetogenic or irritant drugs such as opioids, digoxin, theophylline, chemotherapy agents, NSAIDs
- Frequency, volume, color (e.g., bilious), odor (e.g., feculent), consistency (digested/undigested) of vomitus
- Relationship of nausea/vomiting to any specific recurrent activity, event, position, etc.

Psychosocial

- Effect of symptoms on mood, energy, social interaction, interest in activities
- Relationship of symptoms to psychological causes
- Effect of vomiting on caregiver coping

Processes of Care

Practical

- Reduce odors and place visual stimuli that trigger nausea/vomiting out of direct eyesight
- Optimize air circulation
- Have ample supply of fresh cold water for mouth rinsing and to apply to the back of the neck and brow
- Institute appropriate level of care in order to implement indicated symptom management and support
- Minimize oral intake to the degree preferred by the patient; reinstitute clear liquids as desired after 24 hours of relief from vomiting. Discontinue all oral intake if bowel obstruction is suspected or confirmed

Biomedical

- Basic principles
  1. Obviate and treat the underlying cause whenever possible
  2. Prevention is more successful than treatment
     - Administer antiemetic prior to known triggers of nausea/vomiting
  3. Use nonpharmacological approaches whenever possible:
     - Acupuncture/acupressure
     - Relaxation techniques
  4. The oral route is preferred for prophylactic pharmacotherapy
  5. Use the rectal or parenteral (e.g., subcutaneous) route to initiate treatment for the first 24 to 48 hours to control symptoms; then convert to the oral route if possible
  6. Use combination therapies of mechanistically different agents without similar toxicities for intractable symptoms
- Pharmacotherapy for nausea/vomiting due to:
  1. Delayed gastric emptying/impaired GI motility
     a. Metoclopramide 10 to 20 mg PO q6–8hr; 1 to 2 mg/hr SQ infusion

    b. Add simethicone/charcoal to decrease gas, if eructation is present.

    c. Decrease intrinsic and extrinsic abdominal pressure: elevate head of bed, use loose-fitting and nonbinding clothing

2. Initiation or escalation of opioid therapy

    a. Metoclopramide 10 to 20 mg PO q6–8hr; 1 to 2 mg/hr SQ infusion

    b. Diphenhydramine 25 to 50 mg PO q6–8hr

    c. Prochlorperazine 25 mg PR or trimethobenzamide 200 mg PR q6hr

- Reassess in 3 to 4 days; tolerance to nausea and emetogenic effects of opioids usually occurs, allowing discontinuation of these antiemetic drugs; if nausea and/or vomiting continue(s), assess for other causes prior to changing analgesic

3. Bowel obstruction (nonsurgical care in terminal stage of disease)

    a. Octreotide 150 μg deep SQ (intrafat) 12hr or 300 μg/24 hr continuous SQ infusion, combined with opioid analgesic, titrated to effect

    b. Nasogastric suctioning only if necessary, feasible, and tolerated

4. Vestibular disturbance

    a. Meclizine 25 mg bid

5. Vagal stimulation (bowel obstruction, hepatic capsular pressure, thrush)

    a. Scopolamine 0.3 to 0.6 mg SQ prn (monitor for psychotomimetic effects)

6. Increased intracranial pressure (brain tumor or metastasis)

    a. Dexamethasone 4 mg q8hr and increase as necessary to control symptoms

7. Metabolic abnormalities (hypercalcemia, uremia)

    a. Haloperidol 0.5 mg q6–8hr

- Nonspecific and adjunctive therapy

1. The use of dopamine receptor antagonists (e.g., haloperidol 0.5 to 2 mg PO/IV q6hr prn or prochlorperazine 10 to 25 mg PO/25 to 100 mg PR q6hr prn) in patients who can tolerate the sedating effects is generally effective as primary or adjunctive therapy for most causes of severe nausea and vomiting; these agents are contraindicated in patients with Parkinson's disease

2. The addition of lorazepam 0.5 to 2 mg SL/IV may be useful as an adjunctive agent for control of nausea associated with many etiologies, or when there are nonspecified causes

3. Dexamethasone is frequently used in the prevention and treatment of chemotherapy- and radiation therapy-induced nausea and vomiting, as an adjunctive therapy with dopamine receptor antagonists, benzodiazepines, and/or serotonin (5-HT)$_3$ receptor blockers (see below)

4. Ondansetron (4 to 8 mg IV/PO q6–12hr), granisetron (1 to 2 mg PO q12hr [available as tablets and oral solution 1 mg/5ml] or 10 μg/kg), and dolasetron (100 mg PO or 1.8 mg/kg IV) are 5-HT$_3$ receptor blockers that have been used for control of nausea and vomiting associated with chemotherapy and certain postoperative circumstances; the newest of these

agents, palonosetron, is the most potent and is recommended only as a single 0.25-mg IV dose; these drugs should be considered in those cases resistant to therapies listed earlier

5. Aprepitant (125 mg PO followed by 80 mg PO qd) is a substance P antagonist and may be used in conjunction with other antiemetics for refractory nausea/vomiting resulting from oncologic therapies

6. Olanzapine (2.5 mg PO qd titrating to 7.5 mg qd over 7 to 10 days as needed) is an "atypical" antipsychotic medication of the thienbenzodiazepine class that blocks multiple emetogenic neurotransmitters, including those affecting the following receptors; dopamine, serotonin, alpha-1 adrenergic, acetylcholine (muscarinic), and histamine; this may provide benefit when multiple emetogenic pathways are involved

7. Dronabinol (5 to 10 mg PO/PR q6–8hr) can provide relief from nausea by selective agonism of cannabinoid receptors (CB1, CB2); in addition, the anxiolytic effects may provide antiemetic effects related to psychosocial causes

Psychosocial

- Use imaging and relaxation techniques to control anxiety or apprehension associated with or causing nausea/vomiting
- Teach caregiver management techniques to minimize stress and burden to the extent possible

Goals/Outcomes

- Minimize nausea
- Decrease episodes of vomiting to a maximum of one or two episodes per day
- Reduce care burden
- Reduce social isolation brought on by intractable nausea and vomiting

Documentation in the Medical Record

Initial Assessment

- Frequency and characteristics of nausea/vomiting episodes
- Likely etiology and/or associated causative factors
- Nutritional/hydration status
- Emotional/psychological status: mood, sleep, social interaction, energy
- Physical findings: oropharyngeal and abdominal examination, skin turgor, activity level
- Coping ability of caregiver around this symptom complex

Interdisciplinary Progress Notes

- Description, sequence, and timing of interventions attempted
- Results of interventions, including adverse effects (if any) of pharmacotherapy
- Emotional and physical findings from follow-up visits; caregiver capabilities and coping

IDT Care Plan

- Timing, sequence, and types of interventions
- Schedule of follow-up visits and contingency plans

Recommended Reading

Ernst E, Pittler MH. Efficacy of ginger for nausea and vomiting: A systematic review of randomized clinical trials. Br J Anesthesia. 2000;84(3):367–371

Ezzo J, Streitberger K, Schneider A. Cochrane Systematic Reviews examine P6 acupuncture-point stimulation for nausea and vomiting. J Alternative Complementary Med. 2006;12(5):489–495

Henzi I, Walder B, Tramer M. Dexamethasone for the prevention of postoperative nausea and vomiting: A quantitative systematic review. Anesthesia Analgesia. 2000;90(1):186–194

Tramer MR, Carroll D, Campbell F, et al. Cannabinoids for control of chemotherapy-induced nausea and vomiting: A quantitative systematic review. Br Med J. 2001;323:1–6

Pain

SITUATION: Continuous and/or intermittent pain—defined an unpleasant sensory and emotional experience—that interferes with basic functions, activities, sleep, or social interaction, or otherwise erodes the patient's quality of life to any meaningful extent

Pain is a very common symptom in cancer and other chronic progressive disease states. Along with severe anxiety/agitation and dyspnea, pain that is out of control represents one of the urgent-emergent symptom complexes encountered in the hospice setting. Pain assessment, establishment of patient goals, and treatment plans should be put into place as a high priority and can be best achieved with an understanding that pain is a highly personal experience, modified and amplified by past experience, immediate psychological, physical, and social context, future expectations, cultural norms, and spiritual orientation. Preventative approaches to pain management, rapid responses by the team to calls for help when pain is out of control, and the ability to intervene effectively in a timely manner are key and fundamental measures of quality hospice care.

Causes

Biomedical

- Basic principle: Identify the cause of pain, and treat with the most appropriate intervention:
  1. Cancer-related: Pain associated with direct or metastatic tumor involvement of bone, nerves, viscera, or soft tissues (60% to 80% of all cancer patients)
  2. Cancer treatment-related:
     a. Pain associated with antineoplastic therapy (20% to 25% of cancer patients) such as surgery, radiation therapy, and chemotherapy
     b. Pain caused by noncancer drug therapy, radiation (early and late effects), or surgery

3. Other common painful disorders associated with advanced disease states:
   a. Myofascial pain (muscle trigger point pain with radiating and referred pain)
   b. Arthropathies (joint pains most commonly due to osteoarthritis, degenerative joint disease, or rheumatoid arthritis)
   c. Neuropathies (e.g., HIV, diabetes, peripheral vascular disease, herpes zoster)
   d. Headache (tension pattern, migraine, mixed, other)
   e. Skin and mucosal ulceration
   f. Constipation
   g. Back pain (spinal stenosis, facet disease, spondylosis/disc disease, other)

Psychosocial/Spiritual

- Basic principle: Any amount of pain can lead to a lot of suffering, and any amount of suffering can greatly amplify the pain experience
  1. Pain due to any disease is often greatly amplified by interpersonal conflict or unresolved intrapersonal issues (psychological or spiritual), especially when the pain is a constant reminder of the seriousness of the illness
  2. Pain, anxiety, and depression reinforce each other as complex psycho-physiological interactions that often cannot be readily separated; detailed assessment is necessary in order to direct therapy in the most specific and efficacious way

Findings

Biomedical

- Patient report of pain/discomfort
- Facial expressions or body posturing suggestive of pain (e.g., grimacing, guarding)
- Vocalizations suggestive of pain
- Tachycardia, tachypnea, hypertension, diaphoresis

NOTE: Absence of these autonomic findings do not rule out pain; presence of these findings in a noncommunicating patient is suggestive, especially when repositioning, performing personal cares, dressing changes, etc.

Psychosocial

- Poor sleep
- Decreased coping
- Agitation/restlessness
- Withdrawal from social interaction
- Decreased interest in previous enjoyments (e.g., television viewing, reading, sewing, life review)
- Signs/symptoms of depression, anxiety

Evaluation (Fig. 3.1)

Biomedical and Psychosocial/Spiritual

- Basic principle: believe the patient's report of pain. Because pain is a subjective phenomenon, the caregiver/clinician must believe that the patient's report of

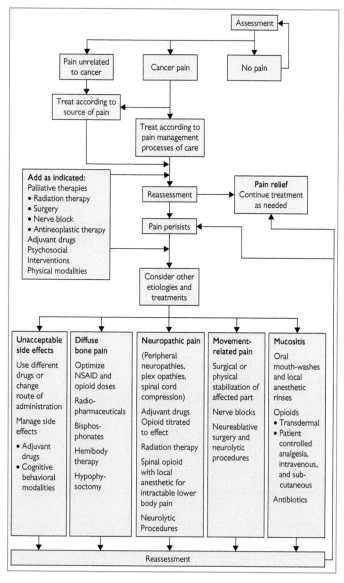

Figure 3.1 Flow Chart for continuing evaluation and treatment of pain (Adapted from AHCPR Clinical Guideline Number 9).

pain is real; objective physiological indicators of acute pain such as tachycardia, sweating, pallor, or affective responses such as facial grimacing are helpful when present but are often absent when pain is chronic or continuous

- Take a careful history, including:
  1. Onset (When did it/does it start?)
  2. Duration (How long does it last?)
  3. Location (Where does it start, and where does it spread?)
  4. Quality (e.g., burning, aching, etc.)
  5. Pain gets worse with …
  6. Pain gets better with …
  7. Pain intensity (measure in able patients using patient's pain rating): measure and record using a standard rating scale (Fig. 3.2; make copies for patient as needed)
     a. Present pain
     b. Average continuous pain throughout the day
     c. Breakthrough pain: frequency, severity, and duration

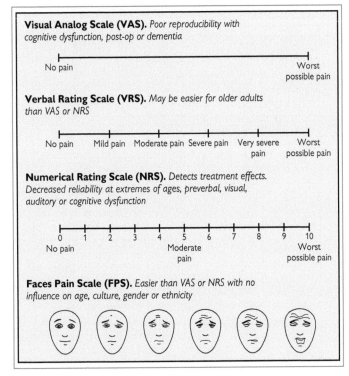

Figure 3.2 Unidimensional pain scales. This figure has been reproduced with permission of the International Association for the Study of Pain® (IASP®). From Hicks CL, von Baeyer CL, Spafford P, van Korlaar I, Goodenough B. Faces Pain Scale-Revised: Toward a Common Metric in Pediatric Pain Measurement. PAIN 2001; 93:173-183. This figure may not be reproduced for any other purpose without permission.

- Incident pain (caused by specific activity or action)
- Spontaneous pain (no identifiable cause)
- End-of-dose failure (pain returns before next dose of regularly scheduled medicine takes effect)

8. Use of a 24-hour pain diary in an able patient helps to identify many factors and effects of interventions (Fig. 3.3; make copies for patient/caregiver as needed)

- Assess the effect of pain on the patient's mood, ADLs, sleep, appetite, movement, toileting, social interactions, interest in life, and previous enjoyments
- Take a careful analgesic history, including prior and present medications, analgesic response (time to onset of meaningful pain relief and duration of action), and undesirable or adverse effects, including frank allergies and gastrointestinal upset
- Perform physical examination and review systems specific to pain complaints

Twenty-four Hour Pain Diary

Patient Name: _____ Date: _____

Time	Maximal Pain 0–10 scale	Minimal Pain 0–10 scale	Medication: name, dose, route of administration	Activities: lying, sitting, walking, eating, toilet, etc.
12 Midnight				
1 am				
2				
3				
4				
5				
6				
7				
8				
9				
10				
11				
12 Noon				
1 pm				
2				
3				
4				
5				
6				
7				
8				
9				
10				
11				

Figure 3.3 Twenty-four hour pain diary

- Review and consider necessity for corroborating diagnostic testing only if the diagnosis is in question or treatment/care plan will be meaningfully effected (e.g., radiograph for suspected pathological fracture)
- Treat pain empirically while evaluation is being completed
- Be as specific as possible in determining the cause of the pain whenever possible (e.g., fecal impaction, bowel obstruction, epidural metastasis, plexopathy, lytic bone lesion, etc.) and institute diagnosis-specific therapy immediately
- Evaluate level of anxiety and signs of depressive mood disorder
- Evaluate for contributors to pain/suffering of a psychological/spiritual nature (e.g., guilt, punishment, abandonment by God, etc.)
- Evaluate patient/caregiver understanding and use of nonpharmacological pain-reducing interventions (e.g., relaxation, imaging, meditation, massage, heat, cooling, music, etc.)
- Reevaluate pain complaints and effects of interventions frequently
- Determine appropriate level of care, based on patient/caregiver response to therapies and coping abilities
- Barriers to good pain management
  - Discounting a patient's subjective measure of pain
  - Difficulty in assessment of the cognitively impaired
  - Myths believed by both practitioners and patients about opioid therapy, including excessive fears of addiction and hastening death
- Patients need to be educated about medication adherence (use specifically and only as directed), physical versus psychological dependence, tolerance, the disease of addiction, side effects, and appropriate dosing of analgesics; many patients as well as family members believe the use of opioids, regardless of indications, will inevitably lead to addiction, creating a deep-seated reluctance to use opioids for analgesia; teaching points:
  - All opioids will result in physical dependence after a few weeks of use, and sudden discontinuation should be avoided as this may cause symptoms of withdrawal
  - Physical dependence is not addiction
  - **Addiction** is a primary, chronic neurobiologic disease characterized by behaviors that include impaired control over drug use, craving, compulsive use, and continued use despite harm
  - **Pseudoaddiction** may occur when there is inadequate pain control, leading to desperate-appearing behaviors suggestive of "drug seeking," but patients are, in fact, "pain relief seeking;" aberrant behaviors around medication use require a differential diagnosis to determine the underlying cause
  - **Physical dependence** is a state of adaptation that is manifested by a drug class-specific withdrawal syndrome that can be produced by abrupt cessation, rapid dose reduction, decreasing blood level of the drug, and/or administration of an antagonist
  - **Tolerance** is a state of adaptation in which exposure to a drug induces changes that result in a diminution of one or more of the drug's effects over time

Processes of Care

Biomedical (Fig. 3.4)

- Basic principles of pain management
  - Use the least invasive and most readily available and acceptable (to the patient/caregiver) agent/route of administration possible. This is usually the oral route
  - Administer analgesics on a regularly scheduled basis, "around-the-clock" (ATC), rather than prn for continuous pain problems; sustained- or continuous-release formulations make this easier
  - Treat breakthrough pain
- **MODERATE OR SEVERE PAIN TREATMENT PROTOCOL**: Analgesic dose titration for pain that is out of control

  1. Initiate pain treatment protocol within 1 hour for residential/home patients and within 15 minutes for inpatients
  2. Immediately reassess and determine cause of pain
  3. Administer breakthrough pain dose of ordered analgesic; repeat in 15 to 30 minutes if ineffective at bringing pain under control
  4. If pain still poorly controlled, increase breakthrough pain analgesic dose by 50% to 100%

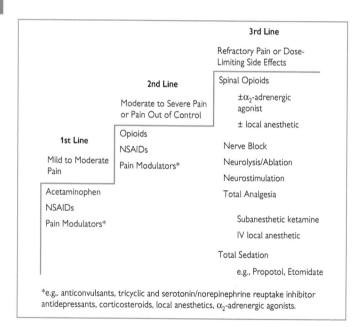

*e.g., anticonvulsants, tricyclic and serotonin/norepinephrine reuptake inhibitor antidepressants, corticosteroids, local anesthetics, α_2-adrenergic agonists.

Figure 3.4 Modification of World Health Organization step ladder approach to pain control. Reprinted with permission from Fine PG. The evolving and important role of anesthesiology in palliative care. Anesth Analg 2005; 100: 183-188

5. **If pain is well controlled,** increase baseline (ATC) dose of analgesic by 50% and continue with newly adjusted breakthrough pain analgesic
   a. Reassess in 24 hours and adjust medication dose based on patient's clinical status
   b. Adjust bowel regimen accordingly
6. **If pain continues out of control** (by patient report of pain out of control or behavior suggestive of uncontrolled pain in noncommunicative patient) 4 hours after initiating protocol, repeat steps 1 through 4 and notify on-call physician
7. If no significant improvement in pain control 8 hours after initiating protocol, discuss with physician and consider pain management consultation
8. If patient is in imminent dying phase, institute pain crisis protocol (see later); notify physician of clinical circumstances

Pharmacotherapy
1. NSAIDs and acetaminophen (Table 3.1)
   a. Indications/advantages
      - Mild to moderate pain
      - Inflammatory pain syndromes, including bone pain
      - Minimal effect on mental functioning

Table 3.1 Acetaminophen and a Selection of Over-the-Counter and Prescription NSAIDs

Drug	>50-kg Dose	<50-kg Dose
Acetaminophen[*†]	4,000 mg/24 hr	10–15 mg/kg q4hr (oral)
	(q4–6hr dosing)	15–20 mg/hg q4hr (rectal)
Aspirin[*†]	4,000 mg/24 hr	10–15 mg/kg q4hr (oral)
	(q4–6hr dosing)	15–20 mg/kg q4hr (rectal)
Ibuprofen[*†]	2,400 mg/24 hr	10 mg/kg q6–8hr (oral)
	(q6–8hr dosing)	
Naproxen[*†]	1,000 mg/24 hr	5 mg/kg q8hr (oral/rectal)
	(q8–12hr dosing)	
Choline magnesium Trisalicylate[*‡]	5,500mg/24 hr (q8–12hr dosing)	25 mg/kg q8hr (oral)
Celecoxib[‡§]	200 mg/24 hr (q12–24hr dosing)	3 mg/kg/24 hr (max 200 mg)
Ketorolac	30–60 mg IM/IV initially, then 15–30 mg q6hr bolus IV/IM or continuous IV/SQ infusion; SHORT-TERM USE ONLY	

[*] Commercially available in a liquid form

[†] Commercially available in a suppository form

[‡] Minimal effect on platelet function (preferred to nonselective and acetylating NSAIDs in patients subject to bleeding or thrombocytopenia)

[§] Reduced GI adverse effects compared with nonselective NSAIDS with short-term or intermittent use

- Supplement with opioid analgesics for moderate to severe pain
- Available over-the-counter in a variety of forms
- Coxibs (COX-2 selective NSAIDs) do not affect platelet adhesion and so are preferred over nonselective NSAIDs when there is a risk of bleeding or patients have thrombocytopenia; short-term use is associated with less gastrointestinal risk

b. Contraindications/disadvantages
- Gastrointestinal distress and ulceration (nonselective NSAIDs and long-term use of COX-2 selective NSAIDs)
- Platelet dysfunction/bleeding (nonselective NSAIDs)
- Hypersensitivity reactions (NSAIDs)
- Hepatic/renal impairment (NSAIDs and acetaminophen)
- Risk of cardio- and cerebrovascular thrombosis with long-term NSAID use (selective and nonselective)

2. Opioid analgesics (Table 3.2, a and b)
- Indications: Moderate to severe pain
- Contraindications
- Allergy or history of sensitivity or dysphoric reactions
- Agonist-antagonist drugs: pentazocine, butorphanol, nalbuphine
- Meperidine (especially in patients with renal insufficiency)
- Precautions: anticipate, prevent, and treat opioid-related bowel dysfunction
- Dose conversions (opioid rotation): Changing from one opioid to another, or one route to another, requires calculation based upon reference to a

Table 3.2a Approximate Equianalgesic Doses of Most Commonly Recommended Opioids Analgesics*

Drug	Parenteral Dose	Enteral Dose
Morphine†	10 mg	30 mg
Codeine	130 mg	200 mg
Fentanyl‡	50–100 mcg	
Hydrocodone		30 mg
Hydromorphone	1.5 mg	7.5 mg
Levorphanol§	2 mg	4 mg
Methadone§	See Table 3.2b	
Oxycodone#		20–30 mg
Oxymorphone**	1 mg	10 mg

* Dose conversion should be closely monitored because incomplete cross-tolerance may occur.

† Available in continuous- and sustained-release formulations lasting 8 to 24 hours

‡ Also available in both transdermal and oral transmucosal forms

§ These drugs have long and variable half-lives so accumulation can occur; close monitoring during first few days of therapy is very important.

Available in several continuous-release doses that last 8 to 12 hours

** Available as immediate- (q4–6hr) and extended-release (q12hr dosing) formulations

Table 3.2b Dosing Guidelines for Oral Methadone

Daily Oral Morphine Dose Equivalents	Conversion Ratio of Oral Morphine to Oral Methadone
<100 mg	3:1 (i.e., 3 mg morphine:1 mg methadone)
101–300 mg	5:1
301–600 mg	10:1
601–800 mg	12:1
801–1,000 mg	15:1
>1,000 mg	20:1

Due to incomplete cross-tolerance and variable potency, it is recommended that when switching to methadone, the initial dose is 50% to 75% of the equianalgesic dose, but be prepared to provide rescue doses of an immediate-acting short-half-life opioid (e.g., morphine, hydrocodone, oxycodone, hydromorphone, oxymorphone) while achieving steady-state doses of methadone (up to 5 to 7 days of tid dosing).

standard conversion table, a safety step reduction and a patient-specific step consideration

- Indications for opioid rotation:
  - Occurrence of intolerable adverse effects during dose titration
  - Poor analgesic efficacy despite aggressive dose titration
  - Problematic drug–drug interactions
  - Preferences or need for a different route of administration
  - Change in clinical status (e.g., concern about drug abuse or the development of malabsorption syndrome) or clinical setting that suggests benefit from an opioid with different pharmacokinetic properties
  - Financial or drug availability considerations
- Guidelines for opioid rotation
  - STEP 1
    - Calculate the equianalgesic dose of the new opioid based on the equianalgesic table.
    - If switching to any opioid other than methadone or fentanyl, identify an "automatic dose reduction window" of 25% to 50% lower than the calculated equianalgesic dose.
    - If switching to methadone, identify this window at 75% to 90% lower than the calculated equianalgesic dose. For individuals on very high opioid doses (e.g., 1,000 mg morphine equivalents/day or higher) great caution should be exercised in converting to methadone at doses of 100 mg or greater per day; consider inpatient monitoring, including serial EKG monitoring.
    - If switching to transdermal fentanyl, calculate dose conversions based on the equianalgesic dose ratios included in the package insert for these formulations.
  - Select a dose closer to the lower bound (25% reduction) or the upper bound (50% reduction) of this automatic dose reduction window on the basis of a clinical judgment that the equianalgesic dose table is relatively

more or less applicable, respectively, to the specific characteristics of the opioid regimen or patient.

— Select a dose closer to the upper bound (50% reduction) of the reduction if the patient is receiving a relatively high dose of the current opioid regimen, is not Caucasian, or is elderly or medically frail.

— Select a dose closer to the lower bound (25% reduction) of the reduction if the patient does not have these characteristics or is undergoing a switch to a different route of systemic drug administration using the same drug.

- STEP 2

  - Perform a second assessment of pain severity and other medical or psychosocial characteristics to determine whether to apply an additional increase or decrease of 15% to 30% to enhance the likelihood that the initial dose will be effective for pain, or, conversely, unlikely to cause withdrawal or opioid-related side effects.

  - Have a strategy to frequently assess initial response and titrate the dose of the new opioid regimen to optimize outcomes.

  - If a supplemental "rescue dose" is used for titration, calculate this at 5% to 15% of the total daily opioid dose and administer at an appropriate interval; if an oral transmucosal fentanyl formulation is used as a rescue dose, begin dosing at one of the lower doses irrespective of the baseline opioid dose.

- Safe storage and disposal: Patients and caregivers should be advised to keep all opioid analgesics and other controlled substances under "lock and key," except for an immediately needed dose of breakthrough pain medication or the next dose of a scheduled medication. Disposal of excess or expired medications is very important in order to prevent accidental usage, especially by children, or diversion. Most tablets, capsules, and liquids should be mixed with dirt or cat litter and placed in usual trash receptacles. Most opioids and other controlled substances should be flushed down the toilet. Opioid patches should be folded over on themselves and flushed down the toilet.

- Driving and functional safety instructions: There are inadequate data from which to make definitive recommendations from available studies. Each patient's circumstances need to be evaluated on their own merits, including disease-related and drug-related impairments that would make driving or other activities dangerous for the patient or others. At the very least, patients (and their caregivers) should be counseled against driving during dose titration and stabilization of opioids and other CNS-depressant drugs.

- Opioid analgesics: specific features, caveats, cautions, and quirks.

Morphine

- One of the lowest cost immediate-release and controlled-release agents due to several generic formulations.

- Some patients cannot tolerate morphine due to itching, headache, dysphoria, or other adverse effects.

- The metabolites of morphine (morphine-3-glucuronide and morphine-6-glucuronide) may contribute to sedation, myoclonus, and psychotomimetic effects.

- Common effects such as sedation and nausea often resolve within a few days.
- Convert to an equianalgesic dose of a different opioid if adverse effects exceed benefit.
- Anticipate adverse effects, especially constipation, nausea, and sedation, and prevent or treat appropriately.
- Oral morphine solution can be swallowed, or small volumes (1/4 to 1 ml = 5 to 20 mg) of a concentrated solution (e.g., 20 mg/ml) can be placed under the tongue for partial mucosal absorption into the bloodstream, although most of the effect is obtained by enteral absorption after swallowing.
- Morphine's bitter taste may be prohibitive in unflavored forms, especially if "immediate-release" tablets are left in the mouth to dissolve.
- Nebulized morphine has been reported to relieve dyspnea (air hunger) in some patients; whether this is due to systemic uptake or due to specific interactions between the drug and receptors within the lower respiratory tract is not yet known; initial dose recommendation: 2 to 4 mg "injectable" or preservative-free MS in 2.5 ml saline for nebulization.

Fentanyl

- Transdermal fentanyl (fentanyl patch): Opioid-naïve patients should be titrated to effective analgesia using short-acting or "immediate-release" opioid analgesics, and then converted to transdermal fentanyl, based upon conversion tables provided in the product prescribing information. See "opioid rotation" above for conversion from another opioid to transdermal fentanyl or from transdermal fentanyl to another opioid formulation. The lowest dose of transdermal fentanyl is 12 µg/hr and this may be suitable for low-weight or frail elderly patients. Time to peak and steady-state blood levels for patients starting the patch is usually 18 to 24 hours. Make sure other rapid-onset dosage forms of an opioid analgesic are available during this time period and for breakthrough pains later on. Although the currently available fentanyl patch is formulated for 72-hour use, end-of-dose failure often occurs as early as 48 hours. Close monitoring of efficacy, duration of effect, breakthrough pain episodes and medication use, and adverse effects is important during the first several days of use and during periods of advancing disease with increasing pain, until a stable pattern of effectiveness is reached.

Instructions to Patients
1. Place patch on the upper body in a clean, dry, hairless area.
2. Choose a different site when placing a new patch, then remove the old patch.
3. Remove the old patch or patches and fold sticky surfaces together, then flush down the toilet.
4. Wash hands after handling patches.
5. All unused patches (patient discontinued use or deceased) should be removed from wrappers, folded in half with sticky surfaces together, and flushed down the toilet.
   - Oral transmucosal fentanyl (formulations: lozenge on a stick, buccal patch, buccal tablet, sublingual tablet, nasal spray): For adults, start

with the lowest dose of the preferred formulation for breakthrough pain, and monitor efficacy, advancing to higher-dose units as needed. Onset of pain relief can usually be expected within 10 to 15 minutes after beginning use. Any remaining partial units should be disposed of safely by following instructions in complete prescribing information; patients and caregivers should be counseled about safe storage and disposal and provided with written information.

Buprenorphine

- Partial mu agonist available in 5-, 10-, 20-µg/hr transdermal patch dose strengths.
  - Initial dosing: 5-mcg/hr patch applied once weekly; titrate up as necessary, or if previously on opioid (up to 80 mg oral morphine equivalent/day) may start on 5- to 10-mcg/hr patch once weekly (medication for breakthrough pain should also be provided).
  - Dose adjustments: generally recommended after 7 days; and not more frequently than after 3 days.
  - Doses 40 mcg/hr or higher may be associated with QT prolongation
- Buprenorphine patch is worn for 7 days; has a well-defined ceiling effect for respiratory depression and respiratory rate rarely drops below 10 breaths per minute (50% of baseline).

Hydromorphone

- Hydromorphone is five to eight times more potent than morphine, permitting analgesic equivalence at lower doses and smaller volumes.
- Hydromorphone can be administered through oral, parenteral (SQ, IM, IV), rectal, or intraspinal (epidural and intrathecal) routes.
- Hydromorphone's relatively short half-life of elimination (2 to 3 hours) facilitates dose titration. Onset of action occurs within 15 minutes after parenteral administration and within 30 minutes after oral or rectal administration.
- Since hydromorphone is highly soluble in water (up to a maximum concentration of about 300 mg/ml), it is particularly suitable for SQ administration, including continuous subcutaneous infusion (CSCI) and patient-controlled analgesia (PCA).
- Hydromorphone is hydrophilic and extensively distributes in the cerebral spinal fluid (CSF) on epidural administration.
- A high-potency preparation (10 mg/ml) is commercially available for opioid-tolerant patients. This preparation is particularly useful for CSCI in patients where small volumes are necessary.
- Side effects associated with hydromorphone are qualitatively similar to those associated with opioids in general and most often include constipation, nausea, and sedation. Hydromorphone may be preferred in patients with decreased renal clearance in order to prevent toxic metabolite accumulation associated with high dose morphine.

Levorphanol and Methadone

- These drugs are useful in selected patients as long-acting analgesics due to their long biological half-lives, making dosing intervals (q6–8hr) relatively convenient. The potential for drug accumulation prior to achievement of steady-state blood levels (four to six doses) puts patients at risk for over-sedation and respiratory depression. Close monitoring for excessive sedation is required by an observant caregiver. Recent evidence suggests that even low doses of methadone may put patients at risk for arrhythmias due to pro-longation of the QT (repolarization) interval. Caution needs to be exercised in patients with electrolyte abnormalities or cardiac conduction abnormali-ties, and when escalating doses of the drug. Nonlinear dose equivalency of methadone requires close attention to dosing recommendations and exten-sive experience.

Oxymorphone

- Oxymorphone is the active metabolite of oxycodone.
- The relative potency between oral morphine and oral oxymorphone is 3:1.
- The equianalgesic dose ratio between oxymorphone extended-release and oxycodone controlled-release in patients with cancer pain was OM:OC 1:2.
- The occurrence of side effects is qualitatively and quantitatively similar for the two drugs at equianalgesic doses.
- Available in immediate-release, extended-release, and rectal suppository formulations.

Tramadol

- Centrally acting analgesic.
- Binds weakly to the mu opioid receptor, inhibits the reuptake of serotonin and norepinephrine, and promotes neuronal serotonin release.
- The WHO places tramadol on step 2 of the ladder as an option for treating mild to moderate cancer pain.
- High-quality studies in patients with noncancer neuropathic pain confirm its efficacy in treating these painful conditions.
- Adverse effects resemble those of opioids, and caution is advised when using tramadol with SSRIs, monoamine oxidase inhibitors, or tricyclic antidepres-sants given the potential for serotonin syndrome.
- Available in immediate-release form, as a single agent and in combination with acetaminophen, and in an extended-release preparation.

Tapentadol

- Tapentadol is a newly approved dual-mechanism analgesic, with both mu opi-oid agonist effects and norepinephrine reuptake inhibition that is believed to amplify the analgesic potency; it is indicated for moderate to severe acute and chronic pain in adults, currently available in "immediate-release" tablets (50-, 75-, 100-mg dosage strengths) and "extended-release" tablets.
- The initial immediate-release dose is 50 to 100 mg q4hr (although a second dose can be given 1 hour after the initial dose), with a maximum dose of 600 mg/24h.
- Associated with significantly lower incidences of nausea and/or vomiting and constipation, and a significantly lower rate of treatment discontinuation and withdrawal symptoms compared with oxycodone.

- Renally cleared inactive metabolite after glucuronidation, so relatively safer in patients with renal insufficiency than opioids with active metabolites (e.g., morphine); no significant interaction with liver microsomal enzymes, so minimal drug–drug interactions.
- Anticipated approval of an extended-release formulation.

Sustained- or Continuous-Release Enteral Formulations

- Several opioids are now available in sustained- or continuous-release form, facilitating compliance and maintaining blood levels between dosing intervals for improved overall control of continuous types of pain.
- Morphine: Commercially available continuous-release pill formulations of morphine last 8 to 24 hours. The continuous-release formulations have similar effects when administered rectally, applied with a small amount of water-based lubricant to ease insertion (no encapsulation is necessary). A sustained-release morphine formulation of pellets in a capsule is available that lasts up to 24 hours but cannot be used per rectum; the capsules can be opened and the contents sprinkled onto a palatable food (e.g., applesauce) as an alternative to swallowing them whole.
- Oxycodone: Continuous-release oxycodone lasts 8 to 12 hours and is available in several dose sizes, starting at 10 mg.
- Oxymorphone: Continuous-release oxymorphone lasts 12 hours and is available in several dose sizes, starting with 5 mg.
- Tramadol and tapentadol are both available in extended-release formulations; see full prescribing information for dose recommendations.

NOTE: Chewing or crushing continuous-release formulations causes them to be IMMEDIATE RELEASE, potentially subjecting the patient to overdosage.

Preventing and Treating Opioid Adverse Effects

- Constipation: Always begin a prophylactic bowel regimen when commencing opioid analgesic therapy:
  - Avoid bulking agents (e.g., psyllium) because these tend to cause a larger, bulkier stool, increasing desiccation time in the large bowel
  - Encourage fluid (fruit juice) intake
  - Encourage dietary regimens (use of senna tea and fruits)
  - For pharmacotherapy, refer to previous section on constipation
  - For opioid-induced constipation refractory to treatment with above interventions, consider the new peripheral opioid antagonist agent methylnaltrexone (see section on constipation)
- Excessive sedation: After dose titration for appropriate pain control, and other correctable causes have been identified and treated if possible, use of psychostimulants may be beneficial:
  - Dextroamphetamine 2.5 to 5 mg PO every morning and midday
  - Methylphenidate 5 to 10 mg PO every morning and 2.5 to 5 mg midday
  - Adjust both dose and timing to prevent nocturnal insomnia

- Monitor for undesirable psychotomimetic effects (agitation, hallucinations, irritability)
- Modafinil 100 to 200 mg PO every morning. This is a relatively safe and effective CNS stimulant that is well tolerated in most patients, but it is relatively expensive
- Respiratory depression: This is rarely a clinically significant problem for opioid-tolerant patients in pain. When undesired depressed consciousness occurs along with a respiratory rate below 8/min or hypoxemia (O_2 saturation <90%) associated with opioid use, cautious and slow titration of naloxone should be instituted. Excessive administration may cause abrupt opioid reversal with pain and autonomic crisis. Dilute one ampule of naloxone (0.4 mg/ml) 1:10 in injectable saline (final concentration 40 µg/ml) and inject 1 ml every 2 to 3 minutes while closely monitoring level of consciousness and respiratory rate.
- Nausea/vomiting: Common with opioids, but habituation occurs in most cases within several days. Assess for other treatable causes. Doses of antiemetics as follows are initial doses, which can be increased as required:
  - Metoclopramide 10 mg PO/IV q6hr
  - Diphenhydramine 25 mg PO/IV q6hr
  - Prochlorperazine 25 to 50 mg PO/PR q6hr
  - Promethazine 25 to 50 mg PO/PR q6hr
  - Haloperidol 0.5 mg IV q6hr or 2 mg PO q6hr
  - Droperidol 1.25 to 2.5 mg IM or IV q6hr
  - Ondansetron 4 mg PO/IV q8hr
- Myoclonus: occurs more commonly with high-dose opioid therapy; Use of an alternate drug is recommended, especially if using morphine, due to metabolite accumulation. A lower dose of the substitute drug may be possible due to incomplete cross-tolerance:
  - Clonazepam 0.5 mg PO q6–8hr may be useful in treating myoclonus in patients who are still alert and able to communicate and take oral preparations. Increase as needed and tolerated
  - Diazepam 2 to 5 mg IV as needed to control myoclonus in imminently dying patients with IV access may be helpful

NOTE: In patients with neuroendocrine cancers, consider serotonin syndrome when evaluating myoclonus; it may exist in a triad of mental status changes, autonomic hyperactivity (i.e.: tachycardia), and neuromuscular symptoms.

- Pruritus: most common with morphine, thought to be due to histamine release, but can occur with most opioids. Treatment-induced sedation must be viewed by the patient as an acceptable tradeoff:
  1. Antihistamines
     - Diphenhydramine 25 to 50 mg PO/IV q6hr
     - Hydroxyzine 25 mg PO q6hr
  2. Benzodiazepines
     - Lorazepam 1 mg SL/PO/IV q6hr

Pain-Modulating Drugs ("Adjuvant Analgesics") (Tables 3.3 and 3.4)

- Basic principle: Always consider the addition of pain-modulating agents when there is a specific pathophysiological indication (e.g., bone pain, neuropathic pain), when there is inadequate pain control with primary analgesic therapy alone, when there is sleep disturbance, or when opioid adverse effects predominate.
- Pain crises *(Table 3.5)*: The first approach to treating pain that has increased beyond the patient's level of comfort is to methodically evaluate the cause,

Table 3.3 Pain-Modulating Drugs

DAILY ADULT STARTING DOSE

Drug	Dose Range	Route(s) of Administration	Indications
Corticosteroids			Cerebral edema, spinal cord compression, bone pain, neuropathic pain
Dexamethasone	2–4 mg tid or qid	PO/IV/SQ	
Prednisone	15–30 mg tid or qid	PO	
Tricyclic antidepressants	10–25 mg HS	PO	Neuropathic pain, sleep disturbance
Amitriptyline			
Desipramine			
Imipramine			
Nortriptyline			
Doxepin			
Anticonvulsants			Neuropathic pain
Clonazepam	0.5–1 mg HS–bid–tid	PO	
Carbamazepine	100 mg qd–tid	PO	
Gabapentin	100 mg qd–tid	PO	
Pregabalin	25–50 mg qd (titrate to bid or tid dosing)	PO	
Local Anesthetics			Neuropathic pain
Mexiletine	150 mg qd–tid	PO	
Lidocaine	10–25 mg/hr	IV or SQ infusion	
Lidocaine 5% transdermal patch: apply to healthy skin overlying painful areas			
Bisphosphonates (see Table 3.4)			
Calcium channel blockers			
Nifedipine	10 mg tid	PO	Ischemic pain, neuropathic pain, smooth muscle, spasms with pain

Table 3.4 Comparison of Commonly Used Parenteral and Oral Bisphosphonates in Cancer Patients With Metastatic Bone Disease

Bisphosphonate Generic Name (Brand Name)	Efficacy in Metastatic Bone Disease	Formulations	Effective Dose
Ibandronate* (Boniva)	Effective by oral and IV routes	IV	6-mg infusion over 1–2 hours q3–4weeks
		Oral (2.5-mg tablet)	50 mg/day
Pamidronate* (Aredia)	Oral route not effective in multiple myeloma or breast cancer; IV route is effective	IV (3-mg/ml, 10-ml vial and 9-mg/ml, 10-ml vial)	90-mg infusion over 2 hours q3–4weeks
Zoledronic acid* (Zometa)	IV route very effective, but no oral preparation available	4 mg/5 ml 5-ml vial	4-mg infusion over 15 minutes q4weeks

* Approved in the United States and recommended by the American Society of Clinical Oncologists (ASCO) for treatment of breast cancer patients and symptomatic bone metastases in men with prostate cancer. Bisphosphonates do not appear to influence disease progression or patient survival; however, they should be considered as a palliative option in advanced disease.

Table 3.5 Analgesic Protocol for Escalating Pain in Opioid-Tolerant Patients

Time (hr)	Treatment
0	Definition of pain out of control: Continuous pain >4 to 5/10 not responsive to current analgesic Rx and distressing to patient
	1. Bolus dose (PO, SL, PR, IV, SQ) 50% of equivalent hourly dose with immediate release dose of opioid analgesic and
	2. Increase ATC doses 50% (notify physician and rest of IDT as soon as time allows)
1	3. If pain still out of control after 1 hour, re-bolus as per No. 1
2	4. If no appreciable change, notify physician for further orders
3 to 4	5. If recommendations by hospice/primary care physician(s) do not lead to adequate pain control (pain continues >4 to 5/10 and distressing to patient): Recommend: 1) opioid rotation; i.e., equivalent dose of alternative opioid analgesic. 2) Parenteral opioid administration (if not already route of administration) with dose titration at bedside
6 to 8	6. If pain continues out of control, contact medical director to consider other pain management options
	7. Consider continuous care versus general inpatient care
	8. Review indications for other approaches to pain control

in order to determine the most therapeutically specific means to treat it, while ensuring comfort as quickly and effectively as possible. Table 3.5 outlines a basic approach to immediate analgesic treatment for patients taking ATC opioid analgesics. The hospice physician and IDT should be notified as soon as possible throughout all phases of treatment to ensure that the most appropriate comprehensive care plan is considered and actualized. The patient's primary care physician and other consulting physicians should be notified in a timely manner, depending on his or her specifications regarding ongoing communication of patient status.

- Most somatic and visceral pain is controllable with appropriately administered analgesic therapy. Some neuropathic pains (e.g., invasive and compressive neuropathies, plexopathies, and myelopathies) may be poorly responsive to analgesic therapies, short of inducing a nearly comatose state. Widespread bone metastases or end-stage pathological fractures may present similar challenges.

- Differentiate terminal agitation or anxiety from "physically" based pain, if possible. Terminal symptoms unresponsive to rapid upward titration of opioid may respond to benzodiazepines (e.g., diazepam, lorazepam; refer to "Agitation and Anxiety" and "Imminent Death" earlier in this section).

- Make sure drugs are getting absorbed. The only guaranteed route is the IV route. Although this is to be avoided unless necessary, if there is any question about absorption of analgesics, parenteral access should be established.

- Neuropathic pain treatment: Recommendations from results of randomized clinical trials:
  - First line: tricyclic antidepressants, SNRIs (e.g., duloxetine, venlafaxine), calcium channel alpha(2)-delta ligands (e.g., gabapentin, pregabalin), topical lidocaine
  - Second line: opioid
  - Third line: topical capsaicin, mexiletine, and N-methyl-d-aspartate receptor antagonists

- Preterminal pain crises that are poorly responsive to basic approaches to analgesic therapy merit consultation with a pain management consultant as quickly as possible. Radiotherapy, anesthetic, or neuroablative procedures may be indicated.

- Consider spinal/epidural opioid/local anesthetic approaches, neurolytic celiac plexus block, or spinothalamic tractotomy. Expertise in these techniques is required; credentials AND experience should be determined in advance of referral.

- From a case-management standpoint, these interventions can add greatly to quality of life and decrease costs if a patient's pain is inadequately controlled by appropriate dose titration of opioid analgesics and adjuvants.

- For truly intractable end-stage pain, parenteral administration of ketamine will provide relief for the patient and ease the great distress that witnessing such agony can cause family and other caregivers who need or want to remain in attendance.
  - BOLUS: Ketamine 0.1 mg/kg IV. Repeat as often as indicated by the patient's response. Double the dose if no clinical improvement in 5 to 10 minutes. Follow the bolus with an infusion. Decrease opioid dose by 50%.
  - INFUSION: Start ketamine at 0.015mg/kg/min IV (about 1 mg/min for a 70-kg individual). SQ infusion is possible if IV access is not attainable. In this case, use an initial IM bolus dose of 0.3 to 0.5 mg/kg. Decrease opioid dose by 50%.

- It is advisable to administer a benzodiazepine (e.g., diazepam or lorazepam) concurrently to mitigate against the possibility of hallucinations or frightening dreams, since patients under these circumstances may never be able to communicate such experiences.
- Observe for problematic increases in secretions; treat with glycopyrrolate, scopolamine, or atropine (see "Imminent Death" section on secretions).
- Dexmedetomidine, an alpha-2 agonist, provides an alternative to ketamine therapy, especially when deep sedation is desired. Use of this agent requires blood pressure and airway monitoring. Dosing: 1 µg/kg over 10 minutes followed by 0.6 µg/kg/hr.

Breakthrough Pain: (Fig. 3.5)

- This is very common in patients with chronic pain and defined as intermittent episodes of moderate or greater pain that occurs despite control of baseline continuous pains.
- Although best studied in cancer patients, there is evidence that patients with other pain-producing, life-limiting diseases experience breakthrough pain a few times a day, lasting moments to many minutes. The risk of increasing the ATC analgesic dose is increasing adverse effects, especially sedation, once the more short-lived, episodic breakthrough pain has remitted.

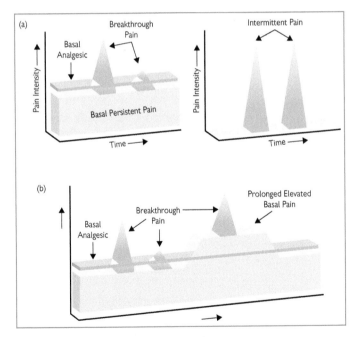

Figure 3.5 (a) Differentiating breakthrough pain from intermittent pain. (b) Differentiating breakthrough pain from prolonged elevated basal pain.

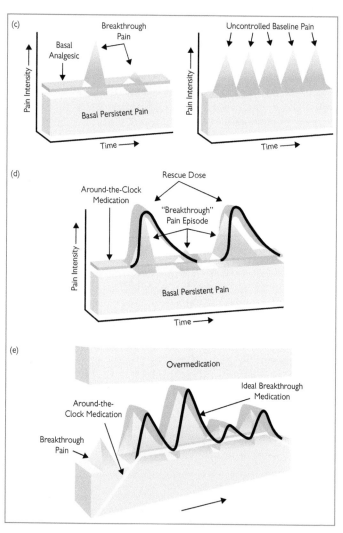

Figure 3.5 (*Continued*) (c) Differentiating breakthrough pain from uncontrolled baseline pain. (d) The rescue dose as a conceptual foundation for breakthrough pain. (e) Management of baseline and breakthrough pain. Adapted with permission from Fine PG. The Diagnosis and Treatment of Breakthrough Pain. Oxford University Press, New York, 2008.

1. Subtypes and treatment
    a. Incident pain: Pain that is predictably elicited by specific activities. Use a rapid-onset, short-duration analgesic formulation in anticipation of pain-eliciting activities or events. Adjust dose to severity of antici-pated pain or the intensity/duration of the pain-producing event. Past experience will serve as the best guide.
        • Conventionally, oral morphine solution or other immediate-release oral formulations of opioid analgesics have been used most

commonly, in order to avoid parenteral administration, but relatively long and inconstant/unpredictable onset times coupled with duration of effect exceeding the typical breakthrough pain episode limits the utility of this traditional approach.

- Oral transmucosal fentanyl (proprietary approved formulations: lozenge on a stick, buccal tablet, buccal patch, SL tablet nasal spray) is an effective, noninvasive means of treating these symptoms in opioid-tolerant patients. IV bolus dosing for patients with IV access may be necessary in those circumstances where oral or transmucosal drugs cannot be used (PCA devices may be helpful).

b. Spontaneous pain: Unpredictable pain, not temporally associated with any activity or event. These pains are more challenging to control. Use of adjuvants for neuropathic pains may help diminish the frequency and severity of these types of pains (see Table 3.3). Otherwise, immediate treatment with a potent, rapid-onset opioid analgesic is indicated.

c. "End-of-dose failure" is the phrase used to describe pain that occurs toward the end of the usual dosing interval of a regularly scheduled analgesic. This results from declining blood levels of the ATC analgesic prior to administration or uptake of the next scheduled dose. Appropriate questioning will ensure rapid diagnosis of end-of-dose failure. Shortening the dose interval to match the onset of this type of breakthrough pain should remedy this problem. For instance, a patient who is taking continuous-release morphine every 12 hours whose pain "breaks through" after about 8 to 10 hours is experiencing end-of-dose failure. The dosing interval should be increased to every 8 hours. If the dose interval becomes too short to make compliance easy, then it is reasonable to increase the dose by 25% to 50%, monitoring closely for therapeutic and adverse effects.

Goals/Outcomes

- Pain out of control (patient self-report of >3/10 pain, or pain greater than patient's acceptable level) is brought under control within 48 hours of admission to hospice
- Pain out of control is responded to with effective intervention within the prescribed time frames in all patients so that no patient dies with pain out of control
- Analgesic adverse effects and side effects are prevented or effectively managed in all patients

Documentation in the Medical Record

Initial Assessment

- Findings from comprehensive pain assessment
- Current pain management regimen
- Patient/caregiver understanding/expectations/goals of pain management
- Concerns regarding opioids
  - Review of systems pertinent to analgesic use: bowels, balance, memory, etc.
  - Counseling regarding driving or other dangerous activities

Interdisciplinary Progress Notes

- Ongoing findings from pain reassessment
- Baseline pain scores
  - Breakthrough pain frequency and severity
  - Effects on function, sleep, activity, social interaction, mood, etc.
- Types and effects (outcomes) of interventions, including adverse effects
- Bowel function, sedation, nausea/vomiting assessments
- Documentation of specific instructions, patient/caregiver understanding, compliance
- Patient/caregiver coping

IDT Care Plan

- Specific pharmacological and nonpharmacological interventions by which members of the IDT
- Contingency plans and crisis prevention/intervention plans reviewed as indicated

Recommended Reading

American Pain Society. Definitions related to the use of opioids for the treatment of pain. 2001. http://www.ampainsoc.org/advocacy/opioids2.htm

Chou R, Fanciullo GJ, Fine PG, et al. Clinical guidelines for the use of chronic opioid therapy in chronic noncancer pain. J Pain. 2009;10(2):113–130

Christo PJ. Cancer pain and analgesia. Ann NY Acad Sci. 2008;1138:278–298

Ferrell B, Fine PG, Herr K, et al, for the AGS Panel on Persistent Pain in Older Persons. Clinical guideline for the pharmacological management of persistent pain in older persons. J Am Geriatrics Soc. 2009;57:1331–1346

Fine PG, Mahajan G, McPherson ML. Long-acting and short-acting opioids: Appropriate use in chronic pain management. Pain Med. 2009;10(S2):S1–10

Fine PG, Portenoy RK. Establishing "best practices" for opioid rotation: Conclusions of an expert panel. J Pain Symptom Management. 2009;38(3):418–425

Fine PG, Finnegan T, Portenoy RK. Protect your patients, protect your practice: Practical risk assessment in the structuring of opioid therapy in chronic pain. J Family Practice. 2010;59(9, Suppl 2):S1-S16

Knotkova H, Fine PG, Portenoy RK. Opioid rotation: The science and limitations of the equianalgesic dose table. J Pain Symptom Management. 2009;38(3):426–439

O'Connor AB, Dworkin RH. Treatment of neuropathic pain: an overview of recent guidelines. Am J Med. 2009;122(10 Suppl):S22–32

Pergolizzi J, et al. Opioids and the management of chronic severe pain in the elderly: Consensus statement of an international expert panel. Pain Practice. 2008; 8(4):287–313

Pergolizzi J, et al. Current knowledge of buprenorphine and its unique pharmacological profile. Pain Practice. 2010;10(5):428–450

Subramaniam K, Subramaniam B, Steinbrook R. Ketamine as an adjuvant analgesic to opioids: A quantitative and qualitative review. Anesthesia Analgesia. 2004;99:482–495

Webster LR, Fine PG. Approaches to improve pain relief while minimizing opioid abuse liability. J Pain. 2010;11:612–620

Pruritus

SITUATION: Chronic or recurrent itching that has a negative impact on the patient's physical or emotional well-being

Causes

- Overly dry skin (xerosis) and moist skin (maceration) are common and easily treated causes
- Contact dermatitis, drug reactions (allergy), fungal infection, and skin infestations should be considered and either ruled out or treated
- Cholestasis or hepatobiliary disorders are common occurrences in many advanced disease states, due to drug reactions, accumulation of bile salts, or obstruction
- Hodgkin's disease, gastric carcinoid, and cutaneous infiltration in malignant diseases cause pruritus
- The majority of patients experiencing chronic renal failure will have this symptom, with up to 60% of dialysis patients experiencing uremic pruritus
- Diabetic pruritus without any associated skin findings occurs in 3% of diabetic patients
- Pruritus frequently accompanies the use of intrathecally or epidurally administered opioids, with a reported incidence between 30% and 100%

Findings

- Self-report of itching or behavior suggestive of pruritus in non-communicative patient (e.g., scratching, restlessness)
- Excoriated skin from excessive scratching
- Skin rash (with or without signs of systemic disease such as conjunctival pallor or icterus, lymphadenopathy, thyromegaly, splenomegaly, or hepatic disease)
- Scratching without relief of symptoms
- Fitful sleep
- Mood alteration (irritability)

Evaluation

- The key to treatment of pruritus (sensation of itching) is identification of the cause; inadequate treatment can lead to excoriation and secondary infection, sleep deprivation, mood alteration (irritability), and generalized discomfort
- History or symptoms as revealed by patient or observant caregiver paying particular attention to the temporal nature of the symptoms, location, and exacerbating and alleviating factors
- Identification of likely disease-related causes
- Physical examination of the skin
- Identification of environment-related causes

Processes of Care

- For xerosis or macerated skin, use lubricating or drying techniques and materials, respectively; using moisturizers and/or occlusives is recommended after washing and drying
- Nonspecific pharmacotherapy can be used until specific treatments take effect or as an adjunct if adequate resolution does not occur:
  1. Sedating agents with some antihistamine activity (H1 antagonist), especially at night, will promote rest and sleep. Titrate choice of drug slowly and monitor therapeutic effects versus undesirable side effects:
     a. Hydroxyzine (25 to 50 mg PO q6hr)
     b. Doxepin (10 to 50 mg PO HS)
     c. Promethazine (25 to 50 mg IV q4–6hr)
     d. Diphenhydramine (25 to 50 PO/IV q6hr)
     e. Cyproheptadine (pediatrics: 0.25 mg/kg/day; adults: 0.5 mg/kg/day maximum dose) starting with a low dose and titrating upward, bid to tid PO dosing (syrup = 2 mg/tsp; tablets = 4 mg/tab)
  2. Serotonin reuptake inhibitor therapy, such as paroxetine 10 to 30 mg PO qd, has been demonstrated to be effective in palliating pruritus not caused by cholestasis or primary dermatologic disease
  3. Gabapentin may be beneficial in patients with uremic, idiopathic, and brachioradial pruritus
  4. Cholestatic pruritus that is not amenable to drug changes or stenting may respond to salt-binding drugs, such as cholestyramine (4 g PO qid), but this drug is generally not well tolerated in very ill individuals. Rifampin 300 to 600 mg/day and opioid antagonists such as IV naloxone and oral naltrexone have been of benefit for patients not able to tolerate cholestyramine in cholestatic pruritus. Additional palliative medications include:
     a. Maalox 15 ml PO q6hr
     b. Methyltestosterone 25 mg SL bid (caution in hormone-sensitive tumors, except in end-stage symptom control)
     c. Ondansetron 4 to 8 mg (IV/PO) q8–12hr
  5. Capsaicin cream or patch is anecdotally reported as being effective, although its use may be limited by abnormal or irritated skin at the site of symptoms
  6. Skin infiltration by malignancies, such as breast cancer, might respond to NSAID therapy, if tolerated. Use maximum anti-inflammatory doses (e.g., naproxen 15 to 20 mg/kg/day in divided doses; ibuprofen 30 to 40 mg/kg/day in divided doses)
  7. Opioid-induced pruritus is usually short-lived, with patients becoming rapidly habituated to this effect; changing to an equally potent dose of another drug (especially a synthetic derivative, because histamine release is common with morphine-like compounds) is one alternative; use of nonspecific pharmacotherapy as suggested above will generally

attenuate symptoms during the habituation phase; patients with spinal opioid delivery systems may benefit from low-dose naloxone infusion (1 μg/kg/hr) or oral naltrexone (12.5 mg PO daily), slowly increasing the dose as needed

8. Suspected skin infestation (e.g., scabies) or fungal infection should be treated with the appropriate primary therapy, complemented by non-specific palliative therapies, as above, to treat symptoms until the cause is effectively treated; inflammatory skin disorders may respond to topical corticosteroid therapy (e.g., hydrocortisone 0.5% to 1% or triamcinolone acetonide 0.025% cream)

Goals/Outcomes

- Relief of physical and emotional distress associated with pruritus
- Prevention of skin breakdown and infection
- Improved sleep

Documentation in the Medical Record

Initial Assessment

- Severity, location(s), and duration/timing of symptoms
- Aggravating and alleviating factors
- Etiology of symptoms
- Physical examination findings
- Effects on sleep, mood, social interactions, activities

Interdisciplinary Progress Notes

- Effects of interventions, including possible adverse drug reactions

IDT Care Plan

- Specific interventions and follow-up plans

Recommended Reading

Etter L, Myers SA. Pruritus in systemic disease; mechanisms and management. Dermatol Clin. 2002;20:459

Gunal AI, Ozalp G, Yoldas TK, et al. Gabapentin therapy for pruritus in hemodialysis patients: a randomized, placebo-controlled, double-blind trial. Nephrol Dial Transplant. 2004;19:3137

Lysy J, et al. Topical capsaicin—a novel and effective treatment for idiopathic intractable pruritus ani: a randomised, placebo controlled, crossover study. Gut. 2003; 52(9):1323–1326

Ponticelli C, Bencini P. Pruritis in dialysis patients: a neglected problem. Nephrol Dial Transplant. 1995;10:2174

Phan NQ, Bernhard JD, Luger TA, Stander S. Antipruritic treatment with systemic mu opioid receptor antagonist: a review. J Am Acad Dermatol. 2010;63:680

Tandon P, Rowe BH, Vandermeer B, Bain VG. The efficacy and safety of bile acid binding agents, opioid antagonists, or rifampin in the treatment of cholestasis-associated pruritus. Am J Gastroenterol. 2007;102:1528

Seizures

SITUATION: Patient/caregiver distress and potential morbidity from uncontrolled seizure

Seizures are frightening to caregivers and exhausting for patients. In addition, they create risk of injury. They should be prevented if at all possible and a plan for immediate treatment should be in place for those patients who are susceptible. These include patients with a preexisting seizure disorder and those with brain tumors or brain metastases.

Causes

- Preexisting seizure disorder
- Structural brain abnormality
  - Primary cerebral neoplasm
  - Metastatic disease to the brain
  - Prior stroke
- Metabolic disorders
- Drug abstinence syndromes (e.g., alcohol, benzodiazepines, barbiturates, baclofen)
- New use or increased dosage of medications that lower seizure threshold in at-risk patients (e.g., phenothiazines such as prochlorperazine, chlorpromazine; butyrophenones such as haloperidol, droperidol; tricyclic antidepressants such as amitriptyline, doxepin, nortriptyline, desipramine)

Findings

- Physical manifestation of seizure varies depending on area and amount of brain involved.
- Possible manifestations include:
  - Frank convulsive motor activity (generalized seizure)
  - Tonic motor posturing (generalized seizure)
  - Focal motor convulsion (limited to one side, or one body part) (partial seizure)
  - Forced eye deviation to one side (partial or generalized seizure)
  - Altered mental status in at-risk patient (complex partial seizure)
- Associated findings may include:
  - Altered mental status associated with disseminated cancer
  - Headache, nausea, spontaneous projectile vomiting associated with increased intracranial pressure
  - "Aura" as a prodrome to seizure activity (e.g., visual, auditory, or olfactory sensory change)
  - Period of altered physical or mental function with gradual return to baseline after generalized seizure

Evaluation

- Review of past medical history should reveal seizure disorder

- In patients who have had seizures, determine seizure risk: how frequent are events, when was the most recent event, what are the characteristics of each seizure, what is the prior use of antiepileptic medications
- Differentiate seizures from other mimics, such as muscle twitching (myoclonic jerks) and alterations in level of consciousness due to nonseizure causes
- If already on seizure prophylactic medications, review schedule, dose, and adverse effects/toxicity/drug–drug interactions
- If "breakthrough" seizure activity while on medication, may want to check blood levels or empirically alter medication regimen per physician consultation
- Determine most appropriate level of care based on patient's seizure history/ risk and current care setting

Processes of Care

Psychosocial/Practical

- Educate patient/caregiver as to importance of prophylactic therapy and acute seizure management
- Assess caregiver's previous experience, understanding, and preparedness for seizure management
- Protect patient from falling and from sharp or hard surfaces
- Do not actively restrain the patient or try to put anything in the mouth; do turn the patient onto a side and lift the chin to help maintain the airway and minimize aspiration risk if possible
- Reorient patient slowly and calmly; Nothing is given to eat or drink until full recovery of sensorium

Biomedical

- Correct readily treatable metabolic or systemic disturbances (electrolytes, glucose, urinary tract infection, fever)
- Re-evaluate medication list for any medications that decrease seizure threshold, as listed above
- Consider pharmacological management: choice based on available route of administration, medication interactions, coexisting hepatic or renal disease, and cost
- Pharmacologic management:

Partial List of Commonly Used Anticonvulsants

Medication	Routes available	Metabolism	Interactions	Cost
Phenytoin	PO, IV	Hepatic, inducing	Many	Low
Valproic acid	PO, IV, PR	Hepatic, inhibiting	Many	Low
Levetiracetam	PO, IV	Renal	Few	Moderate
Phenobarbital	PO, IV, PR, SQ	Hepatic, inducing	Many	Very low
Carbamazepine	PO, PR	Hepatic, inducing	Many	Low

- Acute treatment:
  a. Assess patient safety as above (turn on side, move sharp objects away).
  b. Note seizure characteristics and duration.
     i. Self-limited seizure—supportive care, await return to baseline. Reassess prophylactic regimen and assess for metabolic disarray, infection, fever
     ii. Ongoing or frequent seizure with no return to baseline in between—initial management with benzodiazepine followed by other agents if necessary. Assess for metabolic disarray, infection, fever, and treat if possible and appropriate as related to the patients goals of care
  c. Benzodiazepine choice for acute treatment typically is based on available route of administration. During ongoing seizure, avoid oral route if possible due to secretions, aspiration risk, caregiver safety.

Route available	Medication	Dose
IV	Lorazepam	0.1 mg/kg (typically divided in two or three doses)
PR	Diazepam	0.2–0.5 mg/kg (typically started as 5–10 mg PR and repeated as needed)
SQ	Midazolam	0.2 mg/kg followed by 0.05–0.2 mg/kg/hr

  d. For refractory seizures that do not cease with benzodiazepine administration:
     IV access: Phenytoin IV infusion 20 mg/kg over 20 to 30 minutes in normal saline solution; an additional 5 to 10 mg/kg can be given if seizures persist.
     IV or SQ access, or refractory to phenytoin administration: Infuse phenobarbital 20 mg/kg IV at a rate of 100 mg/min.
  e. In patients with known cerebral tumor or metastases, adjuvant treatment with dexamethasone to decrease cerebral edema may be beneficial (1 mg/hr IV/SQ infusion).

Goals/Outcomes

- Prevention of seizures
- Preparedness of caregiver in the event of seizure activity
- Prevention of seizure-related potential morbidity/injury

Documentation in the Medical Record

Initial Assessment

- History of seizures, seizure control regimen, and effectiveness
- Current disease process likely to pose seizure risk
- Level of understanding/preparedness of patient/caregiver regarding seizures and seizure prevention/control

Interdisciplinary Progress Notes

- Incidence and types of seizure activity
- Patient/caregiver instruction

- Understanding and adherence to seizure prevention plan
- Seizure prophylaxis toxicities/adverse effects
- Reassessment of appropriateness of level of care

IDT Care Plan

- Seizure precautions and prevention/treatment plan and interventions defined
- Follow-up and contingency plans

Recommended Reading

Andersohn F, et al. Use of antiepileptic drugs in epilepsy and the risk of self-harm or suicidal behavior. Neurology. 2010;75(4):335–340

Epilepsy Foundation. First aid for seizures. http://www.epilepsyfoundation.org/about/firstaid/index.cfm

Epilepsy Foundation. Prolonged or serial seizures (status epilepticus). http://www.epilepsyfoundation.org/about/types/types/statusepilepticus.cfm

National Institute of Neurological Disorders and Stroke. Seizures and epilepsy: Hope through research. http://www.ninds.nih.gov/disorders/epilepsy/detail_epilepsy.htm

Schachter SC. Overview of the management of epilepsy in adults. http://uptodate.com/home/index.html.

Skeletal Muscle and Bladder Spasms

SITUATION: Pain and associated distress from spontaneous or incident-related muscle spasms or cramps involving skeletal muscles or bladder

Causes

- Primary neuromuscular diseases
- Spinal cord or plexus injury
- Neuromuscular effects of tumor compression/infiltration
- Infection
- Bladder distention
- Metabolic disturbances (electrolyte abnormalities)
- Immobility
- Indwelling urinary catheter

Findings

- "Charlie horse" of calf, thigh, low back, intercostal, neck muscles most common
- Sense of urinary urgency or crampy, colicky pain in lower pelvis; may also occur during or after voiding
- Bladder pain syndrome manifests as bladder pain, frequency, nocturia, and urgency

Evaluation

- Elicit patient history of bladder or skeletal muscle spasms causing pain during review of systems and physical examination
- Check for dysuria, urinary frequency, feeling of fullness even after voiding, inability to initiate urinary stream
- Timing of muscle spasms in relation to activity, time of day or night, position. Muscle spasm will create nociceptive impulses from the muscle to the CNS; increases in pain leads to increases in spasm (pain–spasm–pain cycle)
- Consider benefits/burdens of electrolyte evaluation based on probabilities of etiology and impact of results on treatment plan

Processes of Care

- Direct primary therapy at cause if feasible and not overly burdensome.

Bladder Spasms

- Nonpharmacological management
- Urinary catheterization:
  1. To relieve a urinary tract obstruction that can't be otherwise managed for a patient with neurogenic bladder dysfunction, hydronephrosis, and urinary retention that can't be relieved by other definitive means, such as with clean intermittent catheterization
  2. To manage urinary incontinence in a patient with a Stage III or IV pressure ulcer and to provide comfort care in terminally ill patients
- Pharmacological management:
  1. Antibiotic therapy for infection (per culture and sensitivities, or empirical use of trimethoprim-sulfa or ciprofloxacin)
  2. Phenazopyridine 100 to 200 mg PO qid (caution about staining from pigmented urine)
  3. Lidocaine irrigation in catheterized patients: add 10 ml of 2% lidocaine to 50 ml saline irrigant, infuse and clamp catheter for 20 to 30 minutes, and then unclamp; useful for short-term relief (less than 2 weeks)
  4. Oxybutynin 2.5 to 5 mg PO q8–12hr prn (caution about anticholinergic effects)
  5. Amitriptyline may be beneficial in persons who can achieve a daily dose of 50 mg or greater in newly diagnosed patients with interstitial cystitis/painful bladder syndrome
  6. Triple therapy with gabapentin, amitriptyline, and NSAIDs for bladder pain syndrome

Skeletal Muscle Spasms

- Nonpharmacological interventions:
  1. Help patient reposition frequently if prone to cramps/spasms; use pillows, bolsters for support and bed rails, trapeze if patient has strength to reposition self
  2. Passively and slowly stretch/elongate cramping muscles with continuous steady force until contraction discontinues
  3. Gently massage with lotion
  4. Actively warm body parts with warm moist towel

- Pharmacological management:
  - Skeletal muscle relaxants are divided into two categories:

    1. Antispastic (for conditions such as cerebral palsy and multiple sclerosis)

    NOTE: Antispastic agents (e.g., baclofen, dantrolene) should not be prescribed for musculoskeletal conditions because there is sparse evidence to support their use and there are serious adverse effects whose potential risks must be weighed against benefits.

      a. Benzodiazepines: Titrate carefully and balance therapeutic effects against sedation and potential memory impairment
         i. Diazepam 2 to 10 mg PO/IV titrated to effect. Repeat based on duration of response
         ii. Alternatively, lorazepam 1 to 5 mg liquid concentrate can be used in patients where the oral or sublingual route is preferred
         iii. Alternatively, clonazepam 0.5 to 2.0 mg PO may be preferable in patients with concurrent neuropathic pain due to its purported pain-relieving actions
      b. Baclofen 5 to 10 mg PO up to tid, based on response and adverse effects (sedation, urinary retention, generalized weakness)
    2. Antispasmodic agents (for musculoskeletal conditions); the choice of a skeletal muscle relaxant should be based on its adverse effect profile, tolerability, and cost (Table 3.6).
      a. First-line therapy for typical back pain syndromes (e.g., low back strain): acetaminophen and NSAIDs
      b. Second-line therapy: cyclobenzaprine or tizanidine; the sedative properties of tizanidine and cyclobenzaprine may benefit patients with insomnia caused by severe muscle spasms
      c. Metaxalone and methocarbamol may be useful in patients who cannot tolerate the sedative properties of cyclobenzaprine or tizanidine; methocarbamol costs substantially less than metaxalone
    3. Quinine sulfate tablets (one or two) PO q HS as tolerated (gastrointestinal intolerance may be dose-limiting) have been reported to be useful in idiopathic muscle cramping (especially nocturnal cramps)
- Intractable spasms may occasionally require special techniques (e.g., nerve blocks) to manage; consult with a qualified and experienced expert if symptoms do not abate or treatment-related adverse effects are overly burdensome

Goals/Outcomes

- Eliminate muscle and bladder spasms whenever possible
- Enable patient/caregiver to be able to palliate muscle spasms quickly and effectively

Documentation in the Medical Record

Initial Assessment

- Frequency, intensity, location, aggravating/inciting and alleviating characteristics and associated signs and symptoms

Table 3.6 Skeletal Muscle Relaxants (Antispasmodic Agents)

Drug Generic (Brand)	Recommended dosage (PO)	Most common adverse effects	Comments	Monthly cost ($)*
Carisoprodol (Soma)	350 mg QID; not recommended for children younger than 12 years	Dizziness, drowsiness, headache; rare idiosyncratic reactions (mental status changes, transient quadriplegia, and temporary loss of vision) after first dose; allergy-type reactions may occur after the first to fourth dose; may be mild (e.g., cutaneous rash) or more severe (e.g., asthma attack, angioneurotic edema, hypotension, or anaphylactic shock); antihistamines, epinephrine, or corticosteroids may be needed	Physical or psychological dependence may occur; withdrawal symptoms may occur with discontinuation; possible respiratory depression when combined with benzodiazepines, barbiturates, opioids, or other muscle relaxants; contraindicated in acute intermittent porphyria; FDA pregnancy category C	72–100 (generic) 590 (brand)
Chlorzoxazone (Parafon Forte)	Adults: 250–750 mg tid or qid Children: 125–500 mg tid or qid; or 20 mg/kg daily in three or four divided doses	Dizziness, drowsiness, red or orange urine, GI irritation and rare GI bleeding; hepatotoxicity (rare); discontinue with elevated liver function test	Avoid use in patients with hepatic impairment; possible respiratory depression when combined with benzodiazepines, barbiturates, opioids, or other muscle relaxants FDA pregnancy category C	15–77 (generic) 180 (brand)
Cyclobenzaprine (Flexeril)	5 mg tid; may increase to 10 mg three times daily	Anticholinergic effect (drowsiness, dry mouth, urinary retention, increased intraocular pressure); rare but serious adverse effects are arrhythmias, seizures, myocardial infarction	Most-studied skeletal muscle relaxant; long elimination half-life 5-mg dose as effective as 10-mg dose, with fewer adverse effects; avoid in older patients and in patients with glaucoma; possible drug interaction with CYP450 inhibitors; seizures reported with concomitant use of tramadol (Ultram), so combination should be avoided in patients with medical conditions that may induce seizures	120–140 (generic) 157 (brand)

				Contraindicated in patients with arrhythmias, recent myocardial infarction, or congestive heart failure FDA pregnancy category B	
Diazepam (Valium)	Adults: 2–10 mg tid or qid daily Children: 0.12–0.80 mg/kg daily in three or four divided doses	Dizziness, drowsiness, confusion; abuse potential	Also an antispastic agent; long elimination half-life; avoid in older patients and in patients with hepatic impairment; possible drug interaction with CYP450 inhibitors; FDA pregnancy category D; avoid especially in the first trimester	11–23 (generic) 184 (brand)
Metaxalone (Skelaxin)	800 mg tid or qid; not recommended in children younger than 12 years	Drowsiness, dizziness, headache, nervousness; leukopenia or hemolytic anemia (rare); liver function test elevation (rare); nausea, vomiting, and diarrhea (rare); paradoxical muscle cramps	Use with caution in patients with liver failure; possible respiratory depression when combined with benzodiazepines, barbiturates, opioids, or other muscle relaxants; less dizziness and drowsiness than other skeletal muscle relaxants; FDA pregnancy category C	275; generic not available
Methocarbamol (Robaxin)	1,500 mg qid for first 2–3 days, followed by 750 mg QID	Black, brown, or green urine possible; mental status impairment; possible exacerbation of myasthenia gravis symptoms	Possible respiratory depression when combined with benzodiazepines, barbiturates, opioids, or other muscle relaxants; FDA pregnancy category C; reports of fetal abnormalities	15–58 (generic) 176 (brand)
Orphenadrine (Norflex)	100 mg BID; combination products are dosed tid or qid	Anticholinergic effect (drowsiness, dry mouth, urinary retention, increased intraocular pressure); aplastic anemia (rare); GI irritation, confusion, tachycardia, hypersensitivity reaction (with high doses)	Long elimination half-life; reduce dosages in older patients; avoid in patients with glaucoma, cardiospasm, or myasthenia gravis; FDA pregnancy category C	110–140 (generic) 162 (brand)

(continued)

Table 3.6 (Continued)

Drug Generic (Brand)	Recommended dosage (PO)	Most common adverse effects	Comments	Monthly cost ($)*
Tizanidine (Zanaflex)	4 mg initially; may increase by 2–4 mg every 6–8 hours until relief; do not exceed 36 mg daily	Dose-related hypotension, sedation, and dry mouth; hepatotoxicity—monitor liver function tests at baseline and at 1, 3, and 6 months; withdrawal and rebound hypertension may occur in patients discontinuing therapy after receiving high doses for long period of time; tapering is recommended	Also antispastic agent; do not use with CYP1A2 inhibitors, ciprofloxacin (Cipro) or fluvoxamine (Luvox CR); caution with CNS depressants or alcohol; decreased effectiveness with oral contraceptives; FDA pregnancy category C	329 (generic) 437 (brand)

Note: The table contains only selected highlights about these medications. All of these drugs may cause increased drowsiness with CNS depressants. Caution is advised when prescribing skeletal muscle relaxants in older patients.

CYP – cytochrome P; FDA – U.S. Food and Drug Administration; GI – gastrointestinal.

* For the recommended adult dosage. Estimated cost to the pharmacist based on average wholesale prices (rounded to the nearest dollar) in Red Book. Montvale, N.J.: Medical Economics Data, 2007.

- Physical examination findings
- Likely etiology

Interdisciplinary Progress Notes

- Types of interventions and effects of therapies

IDT Care Plan

- Instruction in prevention and treatment regimens and specific interventions
- Follow-up plan and contingencies

Recommended Reading

See S, Ginzburg R. Choosing a skeletal muscle relaxant. Am Family Physician. 2008;78(3):365–370

Chou R, Qaseem A, Snow V, et al., for the Clinical Efficacy Assessment Subcommittee of the American College of Physicians; American College of Physicians; American Pain Society Low Back Pain Guideline Panel. Diagnosis and treatment of low back pain: a joint clinical practice guideline from the American College of Physicians and the American Pain Society [published correction appears in Ann Intern Med. 2008;148(3):247–248]. Ann Intern Med. 2007;147(7):478–491

Malanga GA, et al. Cyclobenzaprine ER for muscle spasm associated with low back and neck pain: two randomized, double-blind, placebo-controlled studies of identical design. Curr Med Res Opin. 2009;25(5):1179–1196

Foster HE Jr., et al. Effect of amitriptyline on symptoms in treatment-naïve patients with interstitial cystitis/painful bladder syndrome. J Urol. 2010;183(5):1853–1858

Lee JW, Han DY, Jeong HJ. Bladder pain syndrome treated with triple therapy with gabapentin, amitriptyline, and a nonsteroidal anti-inflammatory drug. Int Neurourol J. 2010;14(4):256–260

Nickel JC, Moldwin R, Lee S, et al. Intravesical alkalinized lidocaine (PSD597) offers sustained relief from symptoms of interstitial cystitis and painful bladder syndrome. BJU Int. 2008;103:910

Skin Breakdown: Prevention and Treatment

SITUATION: Actual or potential skin breakdown leading to patient morbidity and caregiver burden

Causes

- Pressure ulcers resulting from decreased mobility or impaired mental capacity (decubiti)
- Body fluids causing skin irritation/maceration (incontinence, ostomy sites, wound drainage, etc.)
- Itching/pruritus leading to skin excoriation
- Vascular insufficiency leading to ischemia or stasis ulcers
- Tumor erosion or infiltration
- Poor nutritional status
- Friction, abrasion from skin contact surfaces

Findings

- Reddened, irritated skin
- Sources of body fluid/wound seepage
- Nonblanching erythematous skin over pressure areas/bony prominences (e.g., sacrum, hips)
- Partial- or full-thickness ulcers, eschar formation
- Areas of skin excoriation
- Patient may or may not communicate pain.
- Putrid odor from infected wounds

Evaluation

- Elicit patient report of painful, irritating, or itchy areas
- Physical examination of all pressure areas, especially dorsal surfaces of bed-ridden and immobile patients, on a daily basis
- Check for capillary filling over erythematous and blanching skin surfaces
- Identify source(s) of bodily fluids
- Determine cause of itching/pruritus (see "Pruritus" above in this section)
- Consider superinfection of open sores/wounds/ulcers by virtue of purulence and odor.
- Assess abrasiveness of skin contact surfaces (e.g., bedclothes)
- Pressure ulcer stages by National Pressure Ulcer Advisory Panel:
  - Stage 1: Nonblanchable erythema of intact skin; the heralding lesion of skin ulceration; darkly pigmented skin may not have visible blanching; its color may differ from the surrounding area
  - Stage 2: Partial-thickness skin loss presenting as a shallow open ulcer with a red-pink wound bed, without slough; may also present as an intact or open/ruptured serum-filled blister
  - Stage 3: Full-thickness skin loss involving damage or necrosis of subcutaneous tissue that may extend down to, but not through, underlying fascia; the ulcer presents clinically as a deep crater with or without undermining of adjacent tissue
  - Stage 4: Full-thickness skin loss with extensive destruction, tissue necrosis, or damage to muscle, bone, or supporting structures (e.g., tendon or joint capsule); slough or eschar may be present on some parts of the wound bed; often undermining and tunneling
  - Unstageable: full-thickness tissue loss with base of the ulcer covered by slough and/or eschar
  - Suspected deep tissue injury: purple/maroon/discolored intact skin or blood-filled blister from damage of underlying soft tissue due to pressure and/or shear; deep tissue injury may be difficult to detect in patients with dark skin
- Assess and identify severity or degree of progressive/additive risk factors, including:

- General physical condition (good, fair, poor, very bad)
- Mental condition (alert, apathetic, confused, stuporous)
- Activity (ambulatory, walks with assistance, chair-bound, bed-bound)
- Mobility (full, slightly limited, very limited, immobile)
- Incontinence (none, occasional, frequent urinary incontinence, doubly incontinent)
- Nutritional status (excellent, adequate, inadequate, very poor)
- Sensory (pain) responsiveness (no impairment, slightly limited, very limited, absent)

Processes of Care

- Prevention: Caregiver education in the following areas will greatly reduce the risk of skin breakdown and the development of pressure ulcers in at-risk patients (see Table 3.7 and http://www.guideline.gov/search/search.aspx?term=pressure+ulcers):
  1. All at-risk individuals should have a systematic skin inspection at least once a day by caregiver(s), paying particular attention to the bony prominences.
  2. Skin should be cleansed at the time of soiling and at routine intervals, avoiding hot water, using minimal application of friction, and using mild cleansing agents that minimize irritation and dryness of the skin.

Table 3.7 Control of Causative and Contributing Factors

Causative and Contributing Factors	Interventions
Infection	Prevention by using clean technique
	Treatment of infection by the use of topical and/or oral antibiotics
Excessive moisture	Prevention by keeping patient clean/dry (moisture barrier creams, diapers, pads, changing linens, etc.), and consider Foley catheter insertion if appropriate, especially when patient is incontinent; aggressively identify and alleviate any causes of excessive moistures
Shear and friction	Prevention by using draw sheets, not "scooting or dragging" patient across sheets, eliminating wrinkles and crumbs in linens, keeping patient from sliding in bed
	Treatment by quickly identifying and eliminating factors creating shear or friction
Altered nutritional status	Prevention by identifying those at risk with nutritional assessment and taking appropriate action as indicated by assessment; encourage patient to eat/drink if this is consistent with patient goal; provide excellent mouth care as well
Unrelieved pressure	Frequent turning/repositioning, pressure relief devices such as overlay, APP mattress; sheepskin and egg-crate mattresses are comfort measures and do NOT relieve pressure; assess bony prominences frequently for signs of redness, blanching, blisters—take immediate action—do not massage area

3. Use topical agents (e.g., zinc oxide preparations) that act as barriers to moisture and underpads/briefs that rapidly absorb moisture and present a quick-drying surface to the skin.

4. Avoid massage over bony prominences. Current evidence suggests that this may be harmful.

5. Minimize environmental factors leading to skin drying, such as low humidity and exposure to cold; dry skin should be treated with moisturizers.

6. Skin injury due to friction and shear forces should be minimized through proper positioning, transferring, and turning techniques. Use lubricants, protective films and dressings (e.g., hydrocolloids), and protective padding.

7. At-risk patients should be repositioned at least every 2 hours if this is consistent with established goals/preferences.

8. Apply positioning devices (e.g., pillows, foam pads) to bony prominences (e.g., knees, ankles, heels) to prevent direct contact with each other or hard surfaces.

9. Avoid positioning immobile patients with full weight on trochanter (when in lateral position).

10. Avoid uninterrupted sitting in chair/wheelchair by immobile patients if unable to shift weight from pressure points at least hourly. Balance this risk with overall patient goals/preferences.

11. Do not use donut-type devices in chairs.

Treatment

1. In order of most effective (and also most expensive) to least effective, support surfaces to prevent and treat pressure ulcers are:
   a. Air fluidized
   b. Low-air-loss
   c. Alternating-air
   d. Static flotation (air or water)
   e. Foam
   f. Standard mattress

NOTE: The appropriate choice of support surface depends on risk factors, presence and severity of ulcers, ability of caregivers to prevent and treat ulcers, financial resources.

2. Débridement: The method of ulcer débridement chosen should be based on the patient's condition and individual goals/preferences:
   a. Noninfected ulcers should be débrided using dressings (i.e., hydrocolloids, hydrogels, transparent films, alginates, foams) that maintain moisture within the wound bed, supporting the body's own ability to cleanse itself and allowing enzymes present in wound fluids to break down necrotic tissues.
   b. Enzymatic débridement is accomplished by applying topical débridement agents to devitalized tissue on the wound surface.
   c. The simplest mechanical débridement techniques include hydrotherapy and wound irrigation. Safe and effective irrigation pressures

range from 4 to 15 pounds per square inch (psi); the least expensive and most effective devices that deliver pressures within this range are:

- 60-ml piston irrigation syringe with catheter tip (4.2 psi)
- 250-ml saline squeeze bottle with irrigation cap (4.5 psi)
- Water Pik at lowest (#1) setting (6.0 psi)
- 35-ml syringe with 19-gauge needle or angiocatheter (8.0 psi)

d. Sharp débridement is rarely indicated except in patients with a relatively long life expectancy and extensive devitalized tissue with infection; surgical consultation may be required, and pain control should be the highest priority.

e. Heel ulcers with dry eschar are an exception and need not be débrided if there is no edema, erythema, fluctuance, or drainage. Assess these wounds daily, keeping heels slightly elevated and preventing friction or pressure.

3. Wound cleansing and dressings: Healing and prevention of infection is more likely if fastidious wound cleansing is carried out and appropriate dressings are applied. Active cleansing needs to be balanced against inciting pain and aggravating wound trauma. Routine cleansing should be accomplished with minimal chemical or mechanical irritation/trauma:

a. Cleanse wounds with normal saline; do not use antiseptics.

b. Dress ulcers in a manner that keeps the ulcer bed moist and surrounding skin dry.

c. There are no specific outcomes differences for different choices of moist wound dressings, so select one that is most convenient and least costly, such as film and hydrocolloid dressings.

d. Use antibiotic therapy only if fastidious wound care has otherwise failed to control bacterial colonization (exudate and odor persisting after several days of routine wound care).

- Topical antibiotic trial: silver sulfadiazine or triple antibiotic, monitoring for sensitivity reactions or other adverse effects (also see "Bleeding, Oozing, and Malodorous Lesions")
- **No** topical antiseptics (i.e., povidone–iodine, iodophor, sodium hypochlorite, hydrogen peroxide, acetic acid)
- Charcoal dressings may help reduce odor.
- When used topically, metronidazole can eradicate the anaerobes that cause odor.

e. Use appropriate body substance control techniques.

f. Treat pain as indicated in section on "Pain."

- Aerosolized 0.5% bupivacaine or a paste of aluminum hydroxide-magnesium hydroxide may reduce the need for, or dose of, systemic analgesics.

g. For unstageable ulcers, cover with dry non-sterile dressing.

Goals/Outcomes (Table 3.8, a–d)

- Prevent pressure ulcers
- Eliminate adverse symptoms associated with skin breakdown if it occurs
- Minimize morbidity and added caregiver burden by adherence to skin care protocols
- Caregiver comfort with routine skin care protocols

Documentation in the Medical Record

Initial Assessment

- Findings from skin examination
- Risk factors for pressure ulcers and skin breakdown

Table 3.8a Determining Appropriate Goals

Protocol	Patient Characteristics	Goal of Wound Care
H	Serum albumin >3.0 and/or patient eating well; no weight loss in past 6 months; patient ambulatory	Healing*
M	Serum albumin 2.8–3.0 and/or fair nutrition; ≤10% weight loss past 6 months; patient somewhat ambulatory but primarily sedentary; peripheral vascular disease and/or diabetic neuropathy	Maintenance†
C	Serum albumin <2.8; poor nutrition; >10% weight loss; primarily or totally bed-bound or chair-bound; peripheral vascular disease and/or diabetic neuropathy	Comfort‡

*Healing: complete healing of wound is expected.

†Maintenance: wound will not become infected or worsen, but not expected to heal.

‡Comfort: wound will not become infected, may become worse, but patient will be pain-free.

Table 3.8b Protocol H (Goal Healing)

Problem	Interventions
Wound (describe)	See earlier Treatment section
	Assess wound for signs/symptoms of infection, treat any infection with adjunctive antibiotics
	Manage causative and contributing factors, including unrelieved pressure, shear and friction, excessive moisture, altered nutrition
	Dietary consult as determined by nutritional assessment and IDT
	Pain relief, if needed
	If no evidence of healing within 2 weeks after treatment initiated, reevaluate whether healing is a valid goal by assessing causative factors, nutrition, infection, vascular insufficiency; redefine goal as indicated
	If goal remains healing, reassess goal and discuss at IDT at least every 2 weeks

Table 3.8c Protocol M (Goal Maintenance)	
Problem	Interventions
Wound (describe)	See earlier Treatment section
	Dietary consult as determined by nutritional assessment and IDT
	Pain relief, if needed
	If evidence of worsening of wound, evaluate whether maintenance is a valid goal by assessing causative factors, nutrition, infection, vascular insufficiency; redefine goal as indicated; if goal remains maintenance, reassess goal and discuss at IDT at least every 2 weeks

Table 3.8d Protocol M (Goal Maintenance)	
Problem	Interventions
Wound (describe)	See earlier Treatment section
	Pain relief, if needed
	Control odor
	If goal remains comfort, reassess goal and discuss at IDT at least every 2 weeks

- Patient/family's goals of wound care
- Needs assessment (i.e., support services, caregiver capabilities)

Interdisciplinary Progress Notes

- Interventions and instructions given
- Results of interventions and ongoing reassessments

IDT Care Plan

- Specific interventions and instructions to caregiver(s)
- Follow-up plans and contingencies

Recommended Reading

Eisenberger A, Zeleznik. Care planning for pressure ulcers in hospice: the team effect. J. Palliat Support Care. 2004;2(3):283–289

Nenna M. Pressure ulcers at the end of life. An overview for home care and hospice clinicians. Home Healthcare Nurse. 2011;29(6):350–365

Kalinski C, Schnepf M. Effectiveness of a topical formulation containing metronidazole for wound odor and exudates control. Wounds. 2005;17(4):74–79

Zacur H, Kirsner R. Debridement: Rationale and therapeutic options. Wounds. 2002;14(7 Suppl E.):2E-7E

Urinary Problems

SITUATION: Urinary retention or incontinence leading to patient distress or increased caregiver burden

Causes

- Benign prostatic hypertrophy in men
- Prostatic malignancy in men

- Bladder atony
- Urinary tract infection
- Medication-induced retention from anticholinergic drugs (e.g., tricyclic antidepressants)
- Fecal impaction with secondary obstruction
- Kinked, blocked, clogged, obstructed urinary (Foley) catheter
- Patient inability to attend to toileting
- Cauda equina syndrome or other spinal/sacral plexus impairment
- Diuretic effect (especially at night)
- Stroke or other CNS impairment

Findings

- Patient or caregiver report of dribbling or frank incontinence
- Urinary urgency, frequency, dysuria
- Small, frequent voidings
- Infrequent voiding with "overflow" incontinence
- Bladder spasms
- Palpable bladder on physical examination
- Change in normal urine color/odor/clarity (e.g., dark, bloody, malodorous)

Evaluation

- Assess fluid intake
- Review medications (especially diuretics, anticholinergics)
- Systems review with patient, if communicative, including abdominal pain, distention, cramps, bowel movements, change in urinary frequency, volume, color, odor, pain while voiding, etc.
- Abdominal, pelvic, perineal, genital, rectal examination as indicated by presenting symptoms/signs
- Grossly examine urine (volume, color, odor)

Processes of Care

- Try to regulate fluid intake and use of diuretics to avoid nocturnal bladder filling
- Instruct patient/caregiver to have patient void in upright (sitting) position and try to initiate voiding on a fixed schedule to "train" the bladder (i.e., every 4 hours during the day)
- Adjust anticholinergic medications if at all possible, balancing relative benefits and burdens of therapies, side effects, and "competing" symptom complexes.
- Treat urinary tract infection and bladder spasms as per "Skeletal Muscle and Bladder Spasms" earlier in this section
- Consider condom catheter (men) or external pouch catheter (men or women) for incontinence, if no evidence of obstruction
- Teach caregiver care and maintenance of condom catheter system and importance of genital skin care

- Insert urinary catheter (Foley) following aseptic technique.
- Monitor initial urine output: if greater than 1,000 ml, clamp catheter for 15 minutes, and then continue gravity drainage, clamping the catheter for 15 minutes for every additional 500 ml of output
- Irrigate urinary catheters with sterile saline on a regular basis; discontinue if no fluid return, and consult physician.
- Consult with physician if unable to pass a standard urinary catheter with minimal effort.
- Instruct caregiver in care and maintenance of indwelling urinary catheter and drainage system (cleansing urinary meatus, observing for obstruction and signs of infection/inflammation around urethral opening/meatus, emptying drainage reservoir, keeping reservoir below level of the patient's bladder).
- Lidocaine 2% ointment or 4% K-Y Jelly may help decrease pain, burning, stinging, and irritation at catheter insertion site.
- Manually disimpact and initiate bowel protocol per discussion in "Constipation" as needed.

Goals/Outcomes
- Prevent bladder distention
- Prevent pain or additional morbidity from urinary tract infection
- Minimize distress, additional morbidity, social isolation, and caregiver burden due to incontinence

Documentation in the Medical Record

Initial Assessment
- Review of urinary symptoms, voiding patterns, fluid intake, medications
- Physical examination findings
- Effect of urinary problems on caregiver, patient self-image, and social interactions
- Effect of urinary problems on environment (odor, etc.)
- Likely cause(s) of urinary problems

Interdisciplinary Progress Notes
- Specific interventions and results
- Patient/caregiver coping

IDT Care Plan
- Etiology-specific interventions and contingencies with follow-up plan
- Plan for patient/caregiver instruction as required by circumstances

SITUATION: Gross hematuria (visible blood in urine), leading to patient/caregiver distress and/or outflow obstruction from clots

Causes
- Urinary tract infection
- Prostate cancer (men), bladder or renal cancer (men and women)
- Nephrolithiasis (kidney stones)

- Benign prostatic hypertrophy (men)
- Prostatitis (men)
- Benign essential hematuria
- Pseudo-hematuria (non-hematuria-related reddish urine): myoglobinuria, hemoglobinuria, porphyria, bilirubinuria, drugs (phenothiazines, rifampin, pyridium), foods (beets, rhubarb)

Findings

- Patient or caregiver report of blood in urine or red-colored urine
- Blood and/or blood clots in urine or bladder catheter
- Decreased urine output
- Increased bladder/urethral pain
- Bladder spasms

Evaluation

- Evaluate urine for gross hematuria: as little as 1 ml of blood may change hue of urine
- Review medical history, medications (anticoagulants, drugs causing pseudo-hematuria), dietary intake
- Systems review with patient, if communicative, including abdominal pain, distention, cramps, bowel movements, change in urinary frequency, volume, color, odor, pain while voiding, etc.
- If in line with patient's goals of care, consider urinalysis and urine culture
- Abdominal, pelvic, perineal, genital, rectal examination as indicated by presenting symptoms/signs; if history indicates, evaluate for outflow tract obstruction (physical exam for palpable bladder, ultrasound bladder scan)

Processes of Care

- Review goals of care
- If in line with goals of care, and negligible amount of gross hematuria (i.e., not interfering with normal urine flow, no physical distress), reassure patient and caregivers
- If indicated, treat urinary tract infection and bladder spasms as per "Skeletal Muscle and Bladder Spasms" earlier in this section
- If gross hematuria with clots, consider inserting urinary catheter (Foley) following aseptic technique (see above for insertion technique, monitoring urine output, and standard indwelling catheter management)
- Consult with physician if unable to pass a standard urinary catheter with minimal effort; patient may require Coudé (bent-tip) catheter for easier insertion; if still unable to pass catheter, patient may require suprapubic catheter placement by urologist
- Consult with physician if persistent gross hematuria or blood clots; patient may require larger-bore double-lumen catheter (20 to 24 Fr) for easier drainage, or a three-way catheter for intermittent or constant bladder irrigation
- Always continue optimal symptom management for physical discomfort/distress related to etiology and management of gross hematuria

Goals/Outcomes

- Prevent bladder distention, enable adequate urine outflow
- Minimize distress, additional morbidity, social isolation, and caregiver burden due to gross hematuria

Documentation in the Medical Record

Initial Assessment

- Review of urinary symptoms, voiding patterns, fluid intake, medications
- Physical examination findings
- Effect of urinary problems on caregiver, patient self-image, and social interactions
- Effect of urinary problems on environment (incontinence, blood loss, etc.)
- Likely cause(s) of gross hematuria

Interdisciplinary Progress Notes

- Specific interventions and results
- Patient/caregiver coping

IDT Care Plan

- Review of patient's goals of care related to complications of gross hematuria and management strategies
- Etiology-specific interventions and contingencies with follow-up plan
- Plan for patient/caregiver instruction as required by specific circumstances, including when to contact hospice case manager

Recommended Reading

http://www.nlm.nih.gov/medlineplus/ency/article/000483.htm

http://www.nlm.nih.gov/medlineplus/ency/article/003138.htm

Mercadante S, Ferrera P, Casuccio A. Prevalence of opioid-related dysuria in patients with advanced cancer having pain. Am J Palliative Care. 2011;28(1):27–30

Xerostomia (Dry Mouth)

SITUATION: Dry oral mucous membranes, lips, palate, throat, and tongue, often attended by cracking/bleeding oral tissues, is a common finding in patients with advanced disease, causing physical and/or emotional distress to the patient and caregiver

Causes

- Candidiasis (thrush): see "Dysphagia and Oropharyngeal Problems" above
- Drugs with antisialogogic (anticholinergic) effects (e.g., tricyclic antidepressants, opioids, antihistamines, major tranquilizers)
- Radiotherapy to the head and neck region
- Dehydration
- Mouth breathing
- Hypercalcemia
- Mucositis

Findings

- Findings are generally self-evident, but the degree of distress to the patient/caregiver may need to be specifically elaborated by open-ended queries and discussion

Evaluation

- Assessment of patient and caregiver coping and concerns
- Assessment of fluid intake and interest in any type of hydration to relieve symptoms
- Physical examination of oropharynx and skin turgor

Processes of Care

- Tailor therapy to the extent of patient/caregiver concern/distress and specific cause of signs/symptoms if readily ascertained
- Symptomatic treatment can include use of a room humidifier, ice chips, small sips of water, sugar-free citrus drops, and fruit high in malic acid (apples, pears, nectarines) in patients who can control swallowing and whose airway reflexes are intact
- Lemon or lime concentrate in the imitation plastic fruit "squeezers" found in most grocery stores is a low-cost, easy-to-manage aid in symptom management for thirst/dry mouth (stimulates salivation if salivary glands are intact)
- Use of oral swabs with water is helpful, especially to assuage caregivers' concerns or perceptions of a loved one's thirst during the phase of imminent dying; similarly, application of a petrolatum-based lip balm may prevent lip cracking and be of comfort to those in attendance.
- Pharmaceutical care should be directed at treatment of specific causes (e.g., candidiasis) or attempts to minimize anticholinergic drug use if possible
- Cholinergic drugs might stimulate saliva from remaining salivary glands in cases where radiotherapy has obliterated the majority of these tissues:
  - Pilocarpine can be used in doses of 5 mg PO, repeated as necessary, or as a 1% to 2% mouthwash.
  - Cevimeline has a longer half-life and can be used in a dosage of 30 mg PO tid
- Salivary replacement is possible with commercially available "artificial saliva" preparations.

Goals/Outcomes

- Reduction of physical distress to the patient and psychological distress to those in attendance from associated morbidity

Documentation in the Medical Record

Initial Assessment

- Patient expression of excessively dry mouth
- Physical examination findings: signs of dehydration, lip cracking, mouth breathing, oral candidiasis

- Caregiver coping
- Likely cause of symptoms/signs

Interdisciplinary Progress Notes

- Interventions and results
- Caregiver ability to carry out care and ability to cope

IDT Care Plan

- Specific interventions and follow-up plans

Recommended Reading

Haveman C, Huber M. Xerostomia management in the head and neck radiation patient. Texas Dental J. 2010;127(5):487–504

Navazesh M, Kumar SK. Xerostomia: prevalence, diagnosis, and management. Compend Contin Educ Dent. 2009;30(6):331–332

Ngeow WC, Chai WL, Rahman RA, Ramli R. Managing complications of radiation therapy in head and neck cancer patients: Part 1. Management of xerostomia. Singapore Dental J. 2006;28(1):1–3

Wick JY. Xerostomia: causes and treatment. Consult Pharm. 2007;22(12):985–992

Section 4

Appendices

Appendix 1: Palliative Radiation Therapy in End-of-Life Care: Evidence-Based Utilization

Introduction

Palliative radiotherapy is an indispensable tool that can greatly enhance the quality of life in appropriately selected hospice patients with advanced cancer who still have more than a few weeks or months to live. It is primarily used to control pain due to bone metastasis. This form of therapy also can be used to prevent distressing symptoms due to tumor invasion of tissues and organs. In highly selected cases, radiotherapy can allay an "untimely" death from tumor-related hemorrhage, vascular occlusion, or respiratory distress for patients who may not yet have completed their life affairs.

Even in non-hospice environments, it is estimated that about 50% of radiation therapy treatments performed are for palliative reasons like relief of symptoms associated with primary or metastatic cancer. Yet this important form of palliative therapy has not been employed to any great extent in hospice care due to several factors, including cost, inconvenience, and burden to patients, and a lack of understanding on the part of both hospice clinicians and radiation therapists about its utility in this population.

Like all interventions for palliation at the end of life, before embarking upon this form of treatment, the benefits must clearly outweigh risks and burdens. Therefore, hospice clinicians need to understand the potential role for radiation therapy (who, when, what, where, and why). And radiation oncologists need to understand the contextual needs of hospice patients and their caregivers and the system of care under which the final phase of life is being experienced.

Unfortunately, there are few radiation therapy outcome studies that can help direct the care we give to patients with advanced cancer. Much of the practice of radiation oncology is founded upon the personal experiences of therapists, as passed down by their seniors and reinforced through their own practice patterns. Additionally, widely variable approaches are taken to manage similar cases, without well-defined differences in clinical results. These factors prompt the need for critical rethinking in order to provide a basis for rational decision-making so that hospice patients may benefit from the appropriate use of palliative radiation therapy.

Ethical Guiding Principles

(adapted and modified from Mackillop WJ, 1996)

- Palliative radiotherapy should be integrated into the comprehensive plan of care.

- The decision to recommend palliative radiotherapy should be based on a thorough knowledge of the patient's circumstances.
- The decision to recommend palliative radiotherapy should be based upon objective information whenever possible, without adding unnecessary suffering or cost to the patient or family.
- The risk–benefit analysis should include consideration of all aspects of the patient's well-being. The short-term risks and benefits of palliative radiotherapy are more important than those that may or may not occur in the future.
- The decision to use palliative radiotherapy should be consistent with the values and preferences of the patient.
- The patient should be involved in the treatment decision to the extent that he or she wishes.
- Time is precious when life is short. Delays and all waiting times should be minimized. Courses of palliative radiotherapy should be no longer than absolutely necessary to achieve the therapeutic goal. Science, not individual practice patterns or habits, should guide therapy. Palliative radiotherapy should consume no more resources than necessary.

Indications for Palliative Radiotherapy

- Pain relief
- Bone metastases
- Lung cancer causing chest pain
- Nerve root or plexus compression/invasion
  - Soft tissue infiltration
- Control of bleeding
  - Hemoptysis
  - Vaginal and rectal bleeding
- Control of fungation and ulceration
- Relief of impending or actual obstruction
  - Esophagus
  - Bronchus
  - Rectum
- • Shrinkage of tumor mass(es) causing distressing symptoms
  - Brain metastasis
  - Skin lesions
- Prevention of significant functional morbidity and pain
  - Impending bone fractures (long bones, vertebral bodies)
  - Spinal cord compression
  - Superior mediastinal obstruction (e.g., superior vena cava syndrome)

Benefits and burdens

It takes several days to a few weeks before palliative radiation therapy creates significant therapeutic benefits. Therefore, in order for patients to benefit, they must have a life expectancy of at least 2 to 4 weeks. Patients whose cancer pain is not well controlled by other methods can benefit from palliative radiation therapy. Or, when analgesic therapies create dominant adverse effects, palliative radiation therapy also would be appropriate. These are examples of situations when patients *should be* considered for palliative radiation therapy.

Other times, there are cases where radiation therapy appears to be beneficial but when one views the "opportunity costs" involved, it becomes less desirable. For example, the actual time involved for a patient to receive radiation therapy treatment is short, but the "opportunity cost" shows up in the transport time and associated discomfort the patient experiences. Additionally, the patient experiences waiting time and time away from family, loved ones, and the potentially meaningful activities in which he or she could be participating. All of these factors must be taken into account when weighing the benefits versus the costs of radiation therapy.

Many patients *can* benefit from palliative radiation therapy; simply weigh carefully *all* of the factors when deciding on treatment.

Fractionation

Fractionation schedules (i.e., the number and timing of radiotherapy sessions and the radiation dose(s) per session) for palliative radiation therapy are not yet based upon a firm scientific footing. However, there is much evidence (supported in the following paragraphs) that suggests shorter courses of treatment are just as effective as more protracted schedules. An additional benefit of short courses is they incur less acute toxicity in the patient. With fewer trips to a treatment facility, patients also experience less discomfort and have more time to spend in other endeavors. Additionally, palliative radiation therapy can be costly in comparison to the likelihood of the improved outcomes it may offer.

Bone Pain

Where palliative radiation therapy is indicated, there is much evidence to suggest, under most circumstances, that a short course (one to five doses) is as effective as more protracted treatment schedules (10 to 20 fractions) and incurs less acute toxicity. The most recent clinical trials have strongly suggested that single-fraction therapy is very effective for the treatment of metastatic bone pain.

Non-Small Cell Lung Cancer

The Medical Research Council trials in Great Britain compared a regimen of 17 Gy in two fractions with 30 Gy in two fractions, and a single 10-Gy fraction to the two-fraction treatment in patients with poor performance status (i.e., hospice eligible). The short-course therapy (one or two fractions) proved to be as effective as the longer course approach without incurring any greater toxicity.

Brain Metastases

The data for treating cerebral metastases is similar to that for bone disease. The Radiation Therapy Oncology Group clinical trials and European studies suggest that a three-day course of treatment is as effective as a more protracted regimen.

Fractionation Conclusions

Based upon historical and mounting contemporary evidence, one, two, or a few (at the most) fractions represent the most beneficial approach to palliative radiation therapy, when indicated in patients with limited life expectancy. It would be against the interests of any patient to propose, much less institute, a protracted fractionation schedule that is time-consuming, creates patient discomfort, and is costly in comparison to evidence of the likelihood of improved outcomes compared with a brief intervention.

The approach toward minimal palliative radiotherapy has not yet become the norm in the United States, although it needs to be invoked as a standard of care for hospice patients unless new data emerge to the contrary. Disagreement with such an approach should be challenged on the basis of the scientific evidence, and professionalism in all such discussions should prevail, with a focus on what serves the best interests of the patient.

Acute Toxicity

There are several potential adverse effects associated with radiation therapy. Most develop a week or two after treatment, when tumor cell death is at its peak. These after-effects can be anticipated and should be prevented or treated in order to minimize symptoms.

Fatigue

Frequently, patients voice symptoms of fatigue. The cause of treatment-related fatigue during the actual course of therapy is not well understood. It may be an effect of radiation treatment *per se* or the exertion required for the patient to attend such therapy.

A brief course of psychostimulants may be a creative and relatively benign means to treat fatigue. As of yet, use of low-dose psychostimulants (e.g., methylphenidate) has not yet been formally studied for this indication.

Skin Symptoms

The most common finding is localized erythema, which resolves in 2 to 3 weeks after completion of therapy. If there is any discomfort associated with it, unbroken skin can be treated with a topical steroid cream (e.g., 1% hydrocortisone). If skin breakdown occurs, this should be treated like any open sore or ulcer (e.g., decubitus care) in order to prevent secondary infection.

Visceral Symptoms

There is a risk of nausea and vomiting during the course of treatment, and these symptoms may persist for a few days following the completion of radiation therapy. Antiemetic therapy should adhere to usual processes of care, starting with first-line approaches (see "Nausea and Vomiting" in Section Three) and progressing to dexamethasone and then ondansetron or granisetron for intractable cases, as necessary.

Diarrhea may occur shortly after exposure of the intestines to radiation therapy. Anticipation of this occurrence by switching to a low-fiber diet (for patients who are eating a full range of foods) may prevent it. If diarrhea does occur, follow established simple processes of care, prescribing loperamide or diphenoxylate as initial therapies.

Dysuria, Urinary Frequency

These symptoms can occur after brief exposure of the bladder to ionizing radiation. Treatment with phenazopyridine and a low dose of an anticholinergic agent (e.g., amitriptyline 10 mg HS) may provide symptomatic relief.

Conclusion

The sum of the current scientific evidence suggests that palliative radiotherapy continues to be underused in end-of-life care. When it is offered, the frequency of treatment regimens commonly exceeds the likely benefits to be derived, adding greater burden than benefit. An evidence-based understanding and application of its role in symptom management by all healthcare providers and caregivers at this crucial time in patients' lives will lead to an improvement in end-of-life care. As with most therapeutic options, appropriate patient selection and informed consent are the foundation of good care. It is now up to hospice professionals and radiation oncologists to act in accordance with the evidence at hand.

Recommended Reading

Chow E, Harris K, Fan G, Tsao M, Sze WM. Palliative radiotherapy trials for bone metastases: a systematic review. J Clin Oncol. 2007;25(11):1423-1436

Dawson R, Currow D, Stevens G, Morgan G, Barton MB. Radiotherapy for bone metastases: a critical appraisal of outcome measures. J Pain Symptom Manage. 1999;17:208-218

Gaze MN, Kelly CG, Kerr GR, et al. Pain relief and quality of life following radiotherapy for bone metastases: a randomised trial of two fractionation schedules. Radiother Oncol. 1997;45:109-116

Hartsell WF, Scott CB, Bruner DW, Scarantino CW, Ivker RA, Roach M 3rd, Suh JH, Demas WF, Movsas B, Petersen IA, Konski AA, Cleeland CS, Janjan NA, DeSilvio M. Randomized trial of short- versus long-course radiotherapy for palliation of painful bone metastases. J Natl Cancer Inst. 2005;97(11):798-804

Janjan NA. An emerging respect for palliative care in radiation oncology. J Palliative Med. 1998;1:83-88

Mackillop WJ. The principles of palliative radiotherapy: a radiation oncologist's perspective. Can J Oncol 1996 (suppl):5-11

McCloskey SA, Tao ML, Rose CM, Fink A, Amadeo AM. National survey of perspectives of palliative radiation therapy: role, barriers, and needs. Cancer J. 2007;13(2):130-137

McQuay HJ, Carroll D, Moore RA. Radiotherapy for painful bone metastases. Clin Oncol. 1997;9:150-154

Munro A, Sebag-Montefiore D. Opportunity cost—a neglected aspect of cancer treatment. Br J Cancer. 1992;65:309-310

Nielsen OS, Bentzen SM, Sandberg E, et al. Randomized trial of single dose versus fractionated palliative radiotherapy of bone metastases. Radiother Oncol. 1998;47:233-240

Tanner C. Palliative radiation therapy for cancer. J Palliat Med 2011;14(5):672-673

Wai MS, Mike S, Ines H, Malcolm M. Palliation of metastatic bone pain: single fraction versus multifraction radiotherapy: a systematic review of the randomised trials. Cochrane Database Syst Rev. 2004. (2):CD004721.

Appendix 2: Principles of Pharmacotherapy

General Principles

- Maximize efficacy (therapeutic effect)
- Minimize adverse effects (toxicity)
- Minimize cost (conscious and conscientious resource utilization)
- Know, anticipate, and match pharmacokinetics (what the body does to the drug: absorption, distribution, metabolism, excretion) to the specific circumstances of each patient (age, gender, ethnicity, weight, comorbidities, concurrent drugs)
- Know and anticipate pharmacodynamics (what the drug does to the body: therapeutic and potential adverse or "side" effects) based upon the specific circumstances and characteristics of each patient, including history of drug responsiveness and adverse effects

Cost–Benefit

- Use generic formulations when this option exists.
- Use more costly formulations only when there is a specific indication.
- Convenience alone (not to be confused with significant issues of compliance) or personal preferences of the prescriber are rarely, if ever, sufficient reasons for medication selection.

Application of General Principles to Opioid Prescribing Practices

- Use the oral or transdermal route unless there are contraindications
- Contraindications to oral administration: patient is NPO, short bowel syndrome, malabsorption syndrome, dumping syndrome, intractable nausea and vomiting
- Contraindications to transdermal administration: fever, diaphoresis, excessive skin sensitivity, extremes of cachexia or obesity
- Consider the rectal route when oral/transdermal routes are contraindicated, but this is an area where personal issues (patient and caregiver) need to be respected
- Use continuous/sustained-release formulations for continuous (unremitting) pain
- Use immediate-release, short-acting formulations for breakthrough pain or for rescue analgesia (more than three or four doses per day should trigger consideration of upward titration of the long-acting formulation)
- Breakthrough pain doses should be from 10% to 20% of the 24-hour dose of total analgesic (e.g., if a patient is taking 60 mg continuous-release morphine by mouth every 12 hours, the breakthrough pain dose should be about 18 mg [range of 12 to 24 mg] morphine or its equivalent)
- Use alternative or more costly formulations only if there is a specific contraindication to a lower-cost formulation
- If a patient's pain is well controlled on an analgesic regimen at the time of admission, take a thorough medication history, including past reactions/expe-

riences with other opioid analgesics, and change medications only if specific drug-related problems develop

- Use U.S. Food and Drug Administration (FDA)-approved pharmaceuticals and routes of administration (predictable and proven uptake and absorption) unless there is a clinical need for which there is no approved product available; under these circumstances, compounding is justified
  - CRITICAL THINKING AND APPLICATION OF SOUND PRINCIPLES OF PRESCRIBING NEED TO BE THE FIRST STEPS OF EVERY MEDICATION ORDER

Drug Interactions

Likelihood of Drug Interactions Occurring with Commonly Used Drugs			
Drug Class	**Frequent**	**Occasional**	**Uncommon**
OPIOIDS			
Codeine		*	
Fentanyl			*
Hydromorphone			*
Methadone		*	
Morphine			*
Oxycodone	*		
Tapentadol			*
Tramadol		*	
NEUROLEPTICS			
Haloperidol	*		
Chlorpromazine		*	
ANTIDEPRESSANTS			
Tricyclics	*		
SSRIs	*		
MAO Inhibitors	*		
SNRIs		*	
ANTIEMETICS			
Metoclopramide			*
Ondansetron			*
CORTICOSTEROIDS	*		
BENZODIAZEPINES		*	

Recommended Reading

Chisholm-Burns M, et al. Pharmacotherapy: Principles & Practice, 2nd ed. McGraw-Hill, 2010:3–35

Fine PG, Portenoy RK. Clinical Guide to Opioid Analgesia, 2nd ed. New York: Vendome Press, 2007

Fine PG. Diagnosis and Treatment of Breakthrough Pain. New York: Oxford University Press, 2008

Appendix 3: Ketamine Protocol

Background to Ketamine

Ketamine is a dissociative anesthetic agent that has analgesic properties in sub-anesthetic doses. Ketamine is the most potent NMDA-receptor-channel blocker available for clinical use. Ketamine has other actions that may also contribute to its analgesic effect, including interactions with other calcium and sodium channels, cholinergic transmission, noradrenergic and serotoninergic reuptake inhibition and mu, delta, and kappa opioid-like effects. Ketamine also appears to have an antidepressant effect in patients with major depression. Generally, ketamine is used in addition to morphine or alternative strong opioid when further opioid increments have been ineffective or precluded by unacceptable undesirable effects. When used in this way, ketamine is generally administered PO or SC. It can also be administered IM, IV, SL, intranasally, PR, and spinally (preservative-free formulation).

Indications

- Refractory cancer pain, under the following circumstances:
  - "Maximal" titration of opioid (to include trial of oral methadone) with prior opioid rotation
  - Where side effects of opiates have become a limiting factor in further titration despite opiate rotation
  - Where the oral route for other neuropathic agents is not possible
  - Evidence of opioid-related hyperalgesia
  - Opioid tolerance suspected on basis of rapid escalation of opioid dose without evidence of progressive or new disease
- Ischemic, inflammatory, myofascial pain or severe neuropathic pain where there is unresponsive/limited response to standard therapies
- Painful dressing changes (wounds/burns/ulcers) poorly responsive to other analgesics

Contraindications

- Raised intracranial pressure, epilepsy, severe adverse psychotomimetic effects from ketamine or other past hallucinogenic drug use

Cautions

- Hypertension, cardiac failure, history of cerebrovascular accidents; plasma concentration increased by diazepam

Relative Treatment Exclusions

- Recent psychiatric hospitalization, suicide attempt or ECT in past month
- History of psychosis/schizophrenia
- History of recent seizures
- Uncontrolled raised intracranial pressure due to brain metastases or hydrocephalus
- Severe labile hypertension or poorly controlled cardiac arrhythmia
- COPD with associated hypercarbia

Potential General Side Effects

- Although 40% of patients receiving anesthetic doses via IV/SC route have some side effect, there is a very low incidence of adverse effects reported with sub-anesthetic doses of ketamine used for pain control. Potential adverse effects include increased oral secretions, hypertension, tachycardia, psychotomimetic phenomena (euphoria, dysphoria, blunted affect, psychomotor retardation, vivid dreams, nightmares, poor concentration, illusions, hallucinations, altered body image), delirium, dizziness, diplopia, blurred vision, nystagmus, altered hearing, and erythema and pain at the injection site.
- Psychotomimetic side effects generally can be controlled by diazepam, midazolam, or haloperidol/chlorpromazine.

Guidelines for Use (SC/IV or Oral)

- Initiation only by approval of Palliative Care Attending
- Use only on PCCU
- Administration/dose escalation by MD or CRNA (under direction of MD) only
- Nurse in charge and assigned to patient has received in-service on ketamine
- Indications for use met and case has been discussed with interventional pain service +/- IDT meeting
- Full collaboration of interventional pain team
- Accurate weight for patient
- Determine patient's prognosis:
  - If short (days to weeks), use continuous infusion.
  - If longer (weeks to months), consider "burst" ketamine (reduces tachyphylaxis/tolerance issues); oral ketamine (see below)

Required Monitoring

- Monitoring required during initial induction period and then q6hr:
  - Vitals: pulse, BP, pulse oximetry
  - Elicit and record pain score
  - Psychomimetic effects
  - Monitor respiratory secretions
  - Headaches

Continuous IV/SC Infusion Protocol

Equipment

- Small syringes
- Saline boluses
- Ketamine
- Infusion pump available

Adjuvant Medications Available at Bedside

- Diazepam 5 to 10 mg (seizures unlikely at these doses)
- Chlorpromazine 12.5 to 25 mg q6hrs for prevention and treatment of psychotomimetic effects
- Glycopyrrolate 0.2 to 0.4 mg IV/SC for secretions
- Labetalol 2.5 mg q6hrs IV for hypertension/tachycardia

Continuous Infusion Protocol	Time (min from start)	Pain score	BP	Pulse	Other	Medications given
Give 0.1 mg/kg IV/SC bolus of ketamine (e.g., 70-kg patient — 7-mg bolus) Reduce opiate infusion by 50%						
Wait 15 minutes, then monitor	15					
If good response, consider this dose for basis of infusion; if partial or minimal response, give second bolus at double dose (e.g., 0.2 mg/kg)						
Observe for response over 15 minutes	30					
If partial response: Give third bolus maximal dose: up to 0.5 mg/kg, but suggest max 20- to 30-mg bolus	30					
Monitor q15mins and observe duration of effective response (usually 15-30 minutes but occasionally hours)	45					
Calculate mg/hr rate from duration of response (e.g., if 10 mg lasts 20 minutes, then infusion rate is 30 mg/hr)						
Give additional bolus (at last bolus rate) and then start infusion Infusion concentration 1-5 mg/ml (e.g., If 1 mg/1 ml concentration, run at 30 ml/hr)	50					
May be able to discontinue opiate infusion, but have PCA/bolus opiate available q10-15mins						
Reassess in 24 hrs Good control: no change Titration required: increase infusion rate by 0.05-0.1 mg/kg per hour Continue to monitor for undesirable psychotomimetic effects, excessive salivation, tachycardia						

"Burst" Ketamine Protocol SC/IV
Method A (SC)
Initial dose: 100 mg given over 24 hrs
Increase after 24 hrs to 300 mg/24 hrs if 100 mg ineffective
Increase then to 500 mg/24 hrs if 300 mg not effective
Stop 3 days after last dose increment
Method B (IV)
Single 4-hour IV infusion of 0.6 mg/kg

Oral Protocol
Use direct from vial or dilute to 50 mg/5 ml using flavoring such as Kool-Aid to mask bitterness (i.e., add 10-ml vial of ketamine 100 mg/ml injectable to 90 ml purified water, store in refrigerator up to 1 week)
Initial dose 10-25 mg tid or qid and prn
Titrate to optimal effect in dose increments of 10 mg to maximum dose 50 mg qid
Onset of action: 30 minutes; half-life 3 hrs ketamine and 12 hrs norketamine
Maximum reported dose is 200 mg PO qid
If hallucinations, mood disturbance, nightmares, or drowsiness occur, give smaller doses more frequently; drowsiness may also improve with reducing opiate by 25% to 50%

Pharmacy Notes

- Ketamine is miscible with dexamethasone, diamorphine, haloperidol, metoclopramide, midazolam, and morphine
- Ketamine can be irritant; dilute in largest volume feasible of 0.9% normal saline
- Usual dose concentration: 1 to 5 mg/ml
- Inflammation at infusion site can be helped by 1% hydrocortisone cream or by adding dexamethasone 0.5 to 1 mg to the infusion (dilute in 5 to 10 ml normal saline, then add to ketamine)

Recommended Reading

Arroyo-Novoa CM, Figueroa-Ramos MI, Miaskowski C, Padilla G, Paul SM, Rodr'guez-Ortiz P, Stotts NA, Puntillo KA. Efficacy of small doses of ketamine with morphine to decrease procedural pain responses during open wound care. Clin J Pain. 2011 Mar 23. [Epub ahead of print]

Ben'tez-Rosario MA, Salinas-Mart'n A, González-Guillermo T, Feria M. A strategy for conversion from subcutaneous to oral ketamine in cancer pain patients: effect of a 1:1 ratio. J Pain Symptom Manage. 2011;41(6):1098-1105

Cohen SP, Liao W, Gupta A, Plunkett A. Ketamine in pain management. Adv Psychosom Med. 2011;30:139-136

Fine PG. Ketamine: From anesthesia to palliative care. AAHPM Bull. 2003;3(3):1-6

Fine PG. Low-dose ketamine in the management of opioid resistant terminal cancer pain. J Pain Symptom Manage. 1999;17:296-300

Jackson K, Ashby M, Martin P, et al. "Burst" ketamine for refractory cancer pain: an open-label audit of 39 patients. J Pain Symptom Manage. 2001;22:834-842

Slatkin NE, Rhiner M. Ketamine in the treatment of refractory cancer pain: case report, rationale and methodology. Supportive Oncol. 2003;1(4):287-293

www.palliativedrugs.com/book.php?ketamine

Appendix 4: Clinical/Functional Assessment and Staging

Palliative Performance Scale (PPS)

%	Ambulation	Activity and Evidence of Disease	Self-Care	Intake	Level of Consciousness
100	Full	Normal activity, no evidence of disease	Full	Normal	Full
90	Full	Normal activity, some evidence of disease	Full	Normal	Full
80	Full	Normal activity with effort, some evidence of disease	Full	Normal or reduced	Full
70	Reduced	Unable to do normal work, some evidence of disease	Full	Normal or reduced	Full
60	Reduced	Unable to do hobby or housework, significant disease	Occasional assistance necessary	Normal or reduced	Full or confusion
50	Mainly sit/lie	Unable to do any work, extensive disease	Considerable assistance required	Normal or reduced	Full or confusion
40	Mainly in bed	As above	Mainly assistance	Normal or reduced	Full, drowsy, or confusion
30	Totally bed bound	As above	Total care	Reduced	Full, drowsy, or confusion
20	As above	As above	Total care	Minimal sips	Full, drowsy, or confusion
10	As above	As above	Total care	Mouth care only	Drowsy or coma
0	Death	–	–	–	–

Adapted with permission from Anderson G, Downing M, Hill J, Casorso L, Lerch N. Palliative Performance Scale (PPS): A New Tool. Journal of Palliative Care 1996;12(1):5–11. Copyright: Institut universitaire de gériatrie de Montréal.

New York Heart Classification: A Clinical Guide

Stage I heart disease: No symptoms of heart disease [PPS 100]

Stage II heart disease: Symptoms of heart disease at MORE than normal activity [PPS 80]

Stage III heart disease: Symptoms of heart disease at LESS than normal activity [PPS 60]

Stage IV heart disease: Symptoms of heart disease at REST or at MINIMAL activity [PPS ≤50]

Functional Assessment Staging (FAST)

The Functional Assessment Staging Tool is a useful means of codifying far-advanced dementing illness, and it has some prognostic value as a component to hospice eligibility determination under current provisions of the Medicare Hospice Benefit. It was published as Reisburg B. Functional assessment staging (FAST). Psychopharmacol Bull. 1988;24:653–659 and can be located at: http:www.acsu.buffalo.edu/~drstall/fast.html.

ECOG Performance Status

These scales and criteria are used by doctors and researchers to assess how a patient's disease is progressing, to assess how the disease affects the daily living abilities of the patient, and to determine appropriate treatment and prognosis. They are included here for health care professionals to access.

ECOG PERFORMANCE STATUS	
Grade	**ECOG**
0	Fully active, able to carry on all pre-disease performance without restriction
1	Restricted in physically strenuous activity but ambulatory and able to carry out work of a light or sedentary nature, e.g., light house work, office work
2	Ambulatory and capable of all self-care but unable to carry out any work activities; up and about more than 50% of waking hours
3	Capable of only limited self-care, confined to bed or chair more than 50% of waking hours
4	Completely disabled. Cannot carry on any self-care; totally confined to bed or chair
5	Dead

Reprinted with permission from Oken MM, Creech RH, Tormey DC, et al. Toxicity and Response Criteria of the Eastern Cooperative Oncology Group. Am J Clin Oncol 1982;5:649–656.

The ECOG Performance Status is in the public domain therefore available for public use. To duplicate the scale, please cite the reference above and credit the Eastern Cooperative Oncology Group, Robert Comis M.D., Group Chair.

End-Stage Liver Disease

The Model for End-Stage Liver Disease, or MELD, is a scoring system for assessing the severity of chronic liver disease. It was initially developed at the Mayo Clinic to predict death within 3 months of surgery in patients who had undergone a transjugular intrahepatic portosystemic shunt (TIPS) procedure, and was subsequently found to be useful in determining prognosis and prioritizing for receipt of a liver transplant. This score is now used by the United Network for Organ Sharing (UNOS) and Eurotransplant for prioritizing allocation of liver transplants instead of the older Child-Pugh score.

Calculation

MELD uses the patient's values for serum bilirubin, serum creatinine, and the International Normalized Ratio for prothrombin time to predict survival. It is calculated according to the following formula:

MELD = 3.78[Ln serum bilirubin (mg/dL)] + 11.2[Ln INR] + 9.57[Ln serum creatinine (mg/dL)] + 6.43
(Ln = natural logarithm)

UNOS has made the following modifications to the score:

- If the patient has been dialyzed twice within the last 7 days, then the value for serum creatinine used should be 4.0.
- Any value less than 1 is given a value of 1 (i.e., if bilirubin is 0.8, a value of 1.0 is used) to prevent the occurrence of scores below 0 (the natural logarithm of 1 is 0, and any value below 1 would yield a negative result).

Patients with a diagnosis of liver cancer will be assigned a MELD score based on how advanced the cancer is.

Interpretation

In interpreting the MELD Score in (hospitalized) patients, the 3-month mortality is:

- 40 or more: 71.3% mortality
- 30–39: 52.6% mortality
- 20–29: 19.6% mortality
- 10–19: 6.0% mortality
- <9: 1.9% mortality

Index

X